Objectives
for Care

Specifying Standards
for Clinical Nursing

Second Edition

Objectives
for Care

Specifying Standards
for Clinical Nursing

Second Edition

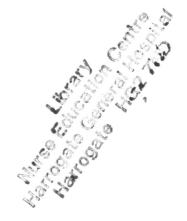

Edited by
Gillian D. Snowley
MEd BSc(Hons) DN(Lond) RGN RNT
Deputy Director
Humberside College of Health
Hull, England

Peter J. Nicklin
MBA MEd DipEd(Lond) RGN RMN RNT
Director of York and Scarborough College
York, England

John A. Birch
OBE PhD MEd RGN RNT
Director of Quality Assurance
and Executive Director
North Lincolnshire Health Authority
Lincoln, England

Wolfe Publishing Ltd

Published by
Wolfe Publishing Ltd
Brook House
2–16 Torrington Place
London WC1E 7LT

Printed by Antony Rowe Ltd, Chippenham, Wiltshire

ISBN 0 7234 1809 8

For full details of all Wolfe Nursing titles please write to:
Wolfe Publishing Ltd, Brook House, 2–16 Torrington Place, London
WC1E 7LT, England.

Contents

Acknowledgements

The editors wish to extend their appreciation to all the contributors to the first edition of this book whose endeavour, co-operation and hard work have made this venture possible. Those contributors were as follows: Sharon Antcliffe, Sandra Blow, Michael J. Cook, Nancy Coupland, E. Margaret Danby, Moonee Gungaphul, Laura Hammond, Christopher Hanger, Norma Haynes, Christine Lawes, Lorna Laws, Kathleen Lister, John Marsden, Josie Marshall, John W. Orchard, Janet E. Palmer, Mike Popat, Colin Raby, M. Ann Rodger, Helen Scott-South, Joan Tong, Jean E. Toyne and Jessie R. Worland.

Foreword

Having been slightly involved in some of the initial work which led to the first edition of this book, I am delighted to contribute this Foreword to the second edition of *Objectives for Care*.

The idea of setting clear, research and practice related standards for care is now a comparatively well-known, but not universally well-achieved, concept within the Health Service.

At the same time when the first edition of this book was published such a venture was rare, not to say avant-garde. It says much for the validity of the concept that health service management as a whole has now caught up with the need to set and define standards for its various services, not least in order to set contracts and costs which are founded upon clear standards of practice and performance.

The word 'objective' has several meanings, two of which are particularly apt when applied to the title and content of this book. As an adjective it means that the subject under discussion is related to facts, impartially assessed and judged, and relying upon sound evidence. As a noun it relates to an aim or purpose which is to be achieved.

These clearly expressed standards of practice are based upon sound evidence, clinical expertise, and relevant and updated research. But such quality of care is not provided by individuals working alone. The care of patients is delivered within a complex and frequently changing organisation of people, premises, and equipment. Policies of care are changing, patient turnover increasing, student nurses come and go at regular intervals, new staff are employed and part-time or agency staff may find themselves working in a variety of patient specialities at different times.

In this situation it is vital that clearly defined and agreed standards of care are readily available, thus enabling all staff to play their part in the overall performance of the ward or team. Under pressure it is easy to fall into providing routine physical care related primarily to the diagnostic group of the patient rather than the total care which encompasses the personal, emotional and spiritual needs and which is supremely the role of the nurse. There is a danger that the drive for efficiency (which is an important component of quality) may override the equally important dimensions of effectiveness, acceptability and appropriateness.

As an organisation becomes more complex, the need for sound organisational guidelines which ensure the co-ordination and consistency of its practice and performance increases. That need is met fully and concisely in the contents of this book, which span the concepts of both the quality cycle and the nursing process.

Aims are clearly defined, together with information on the assessment, planning and implementation of the care needed to achieve the stated aims. The section on evaluation provides a basis for care audit, and (refreshingly) really does represent a proper application of the term 'outcome' which is defined by Donabedian (1980) as:

> 'a change in the patient's current and future health (including physical, psychological and social health) and behaviour that can be attributed to antecedent care.'

Thus this book initially designed for the use of practitioners and students, mentors and ward managers now extends its relevance and meets a wider need. Its clear objectives and definitions, its applicability to patients in all care specialities and settings, provides a basis for defining contract standards which can be used by general managers and business planners, purchasers and providers of health care. It should also be used in accreditation systems, and for audit by both professional and consumer groups.

The new section on audit is particularly timely and would be of assistance to other professional groups who are now embarking on the task of making quality assurance real rather than rhetorical.

Reference
Donabedian, A. (1980) *The Definition of Quality Assurance and Approaches to its Measurement*, AnnArbor, Health Administration Press.

Jean A. Ball, Senior Teaching Fellow
Nuffield Institute for Health Services Studies,
University of Leeds.

Introduction

The primary purpose of the first edition of *Objectives for Care* (1987) was to assist nurses to prescribe and evaluate nursing actions by formulating objectives that would form the basis for 'acceptable standards of care'. Whilst the objectives for care have not changed substantially since the publication of the first edition of this book, the managerial and organisational context in which nursing care is delivered has been radically reformed. This second edition briefly outlines the changing context of care delivery and describes the utilisation of objectives for care in the process of **Auditing Nursing Services**.

Quality

The central concern of *Working for Patients* (Department of Health, 1989a) and *Caring for People* (Department of Health 1989b) is to provide patients and clients with better quality care and services. Quality is, however, a notoriously difficult concept to describe and define. Charles Shaw in *Introducing Quality Assurance* (1986) suggests that 'watertight definitions of quality and related words are too elusive to merit the time of practical people' and proceeds to identify the essential 'elements' of quality:

- **Appropriateness**: the service or procedure is what the population or individual actually needs.
- **Equity**: a fair share for all the population.
- **Accessibility**: services are not compromised by undue limits of time or distance.
- **Effectiveness**: achieving the intended benefit for the individual and for the population.
- **Acceptability**: services are provided such as to satisfy the reasonable expectations of patients, providers and the community.

1

- **Efficiency**: resources are not wasted on one service or patient to the detriment of another.

Shaw asserts that of these the key element is **Appropriateness**. For example, a post-operative patient may be nursed at rest in bed and routine observations conducted competently, but if the patient is capable of mobilization and the measurement and recording of temperature, pulse and respiration are 'ritual' rather than required this case is inappropriate. If care is inappropriate it exacts a high price from the patient and a cash limited service; in short—quality is compromised. Additionally, good quality does not necessarily mean the highest possible quality of care. It means a predictable degree of uniformity and dependability and *agreed standard of care, appropriate to the needs of the patient*. It is with the 'element' of appropriateness that this book is particularly concerned.

Audit of Nursing Services

The first edition of this book placed *objectives for care* in the context of what was then described as the 'nursing process'. This edition seeks to locate clinical care objectives in the broader context of *Nursing Audit*. The NHS Management Executive (1991) defines Nursing Audit as:

> 'part of the cycle of quality assurance. It incorporates the systematic and critical analysis by nurses, midwives and health visitors, in conjunction with other staff, of the planning, delivery and evaluation of Nursing and Midwifery care, in terms of their use of resources and outcomes for patients and clients and introduces appropriate change in response to that analysis'.

The Audit of Nursing Services is, therefore, a comprehensive construct not soley confined to the delivery of direct clinical care but embraces issues relating to:

- **Workload management**: identifying and prioritising what care is required.
- **Deployment**: establishing the skills that are required and which grade of staff will most efficiently deliver the required care.
- **Personnel management**: recruitment, selection, training, development and retention of staff to deliver care.
- **Organisational arrangements**: development, implementation and monitoring of policies that inform the delivery of care.
- **Environment and support**: availability, cost and delivery of supplies and services required to enable the prescribed care to be given.

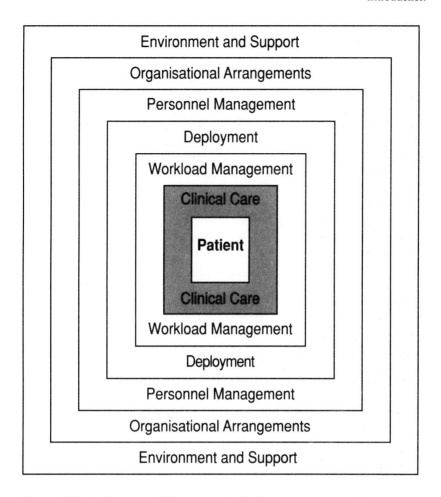

Figure 1. The 'audit square'. (Courtesy of Dr A. Kamal, North Lincolnshire Health.)

This interactive relationship is illustrated in the framework for Audit proposed by the NHS Management Executive (1991) (*Figure 1*).

The methodical and analytical audit of each of these dynamically related areas will enable clinical nurses and their managers to provide cost effective care of appropriate quality, and in doing so ensures that nurses meet their professional obligation to the individual patient and that the 'provider' unit satisfies its contractual obligations to the 'purchasers' of care.

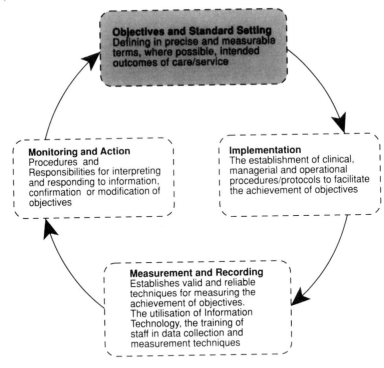

Figure 2. The 'audit cycle'. (Courtesy of Mr S. Hoey.)

The audit process

Each of the six areas illustrated in *Figure 1* can be audited using a four stage cyclical process (*Figure 2*).

Objectives and standards

The objectives contained in the subsequent chapters of this book provide a focus for formulating standards of clinical care employing Henderson's (1969) classification of the components of nursing care. Whilst objectives describe, in general terms, the proposed purposes of care they do not specify in measurable terms what standard of care should be delivered. The development of *standards* is the first phase of the **Audit Cycle**.

Crow (1981) asserts that 'standards is some measure or measures by which nursing care may be judged or compared and where measures used are agreed upon by common consent.' The precision of this definition does however conceal the complexity of prioritising and framing standards. In other words, are all standards of equal importance and are all standards amenable to precise description and measurement; more simply do all standards have the same essential characteristics? The standards declared in *The Patients Charter* (Department of Health, 1991) illustrate this complexity of prioritising and framing standards:

. . . the NHS will be aiming to provide for you:
- an emergency ambulance should arrive within 14 minutes in an urban area . . .
- respect for privacy, dignity and religious and cultural beliefs.

These standards, which are both important, clearly have quite different characteristics. The achievement of the first can be judged with the use of a stop watch. Judging the accomplishment of the second may be in part reliant on intuition and feelings. In the pursuit of 'scientific measurement' there can be a tendency to become preoccupied with those standards which are amenable to precise measurement at the expense of equally important standards whose description and attainment is more illusive because of their complexity. Alison Kitson (1987) in her authoritative discussion on this issue asserts that raising standards 'has little to do with static protocols and rigid systems; rather it has more to do with stout hearts and gut reactions . . . the search for what is best for a person in need is always more complex than such simple descriptions of standard helping procedures imply'. Kitson concludes her argument with the assertion that the 'intuitive' must be linked to the 'scientific' if the profession is to meet its obligations to society.

In the preparation of 'objectives for care' the contributors have been confronted with precisely the same issue. The following two examples of objectives illustrate this point:

- **Communication objective** (page 29)—'provide a sufficiently relaxed atmosphere for the person to communicate freely and to inspire confidence'.

is an important objective and its achievement could be confirmed through a 'Patient Satisfaction Survey', or failure revealed by a complaint: however agreeing a precise standard for this objective would be extremely difficult. Conversely,

- **Mobility objective** (page 24)—assess the person's risk for the development of pressure sores.

also an important objective, could be expressed as a precise and measurable standard, for example:

- **Standard**—all patients' risk of developing pressure sores will be assessed on the Waterlow Scale every 24 hours.

Whilst it is possible and useful to formulate generalised objectives for care, which have a broad application, the development of standards is situation and client group specific. In refining objectives for care into specific and measurable standards the following are key issues:

- Is the standard acceptable to patients/clients?
- Is the standard acceptable to those delivering care?
- Is the standard 'owned' and easily understood by all participating in care delivery?
- Is the standard affordable and achievable?

Area	Clinical Care				Sheet		
Category	Therapeutic Care				A	2	1
Issue	Resting and Sleeping for Patients (pp 46–48)						
Version	1.0	Revision date			Revised by		

Objective
To minimise patients' distress, irritations and discomfort caused by lack of sleep.

Standard(s)
- All patients will enjoy a sleep pattern which is as close as possible to their normal routine.
- Disturbed and inadequate sleep patterns will be restored to normal for each individual whenever possible.

Implementation
- Staff are educated in general aspects of sleep and factors which disturb normal sleep, skills of assessment and planning for adequate sleep in hospital.
- Sleep standards are communicated to all staff, patients and relatives.
- Care routines are flexible to accommodate individual sleep programmes, including pre-sleep rituals.
- Pain relieving measures and therapeutic interventions for comfort are provided whenever necessary.
- Physical standards in the environment and staff activities are altered, when necessary, to reduce noise and interference.
- Patients and relatives are made aware of opportunities for relatives to stay overnight.
- All primary nurses are responsible for reporting and supplying sleep audit data.

Measuring and Recording
- Observation and interviews with patients, daily reporting and appropriate alteration of care plans will be employed.
- The views of random samples of patients and/or their relatives will be obtained by confidential questionnaire every 3 months.
- The views of a cross section of care staff (all professions) will be sought every 3 months.

Monitoring and Action
- Care routines are altered, if necessary, in accordance with patient satisfaction surveys.
- Primary nurses are responsible for making procedural alterations for their named patients.

Cross-refs				Data Source(s)	

Figure 3. Use of 'Objectives for Care' in a Clinical Care Audit (NHS Management Executive, 1991).

Establishing priorities for Clinical Care Audit will be significantly influenced by local concerns and aspirations. Consequently it is not possible to prescribe those areas of care that are most suitable or appropriate for audit. *Figures 3* and *4* illustrate the use of 'Objectives for Care' in Clinical Care Audit: these specimen audit protocols are based on the NHS Management Executive (1991) guidance and reveal the four stages of the Audit Cycle.

Area	Clinical Care			Sheet		
Category	Supportive Care			A	2	1
Issue	Religion (pp 49–51)					
Version	1.0	Revision date		Revised by		

Objective
To allow complete freedom to every patient to practise their religion.

Standard(s)
- Facilities will always be available for patients to continue with worship or other religious activity.
- Patients and/or their families will be able to carry out specific religious rites and customs associated with feeding, hygiene, dress and prayer.
- Clergy and leaders of ethnic religious groups will have 24 hour access to patients, at the request of the patient.
- Whenever appropriate, specific rites and customs will be carried out following the death of a patient.

Implementation
- On admission to care all patients will be asked about their requirements for religious activity, if any.
- All care staff are educated in the specific aspects of religious practices of Christians, Jews, Moslems, Hindus (. . . and any other).
- All staff are aware of the procedure to be followed if a patient refuses medical treatment for religious reasons.
- Primary nurses are responsible for reporting and supplying audit data.

Measuring and Recording
- Regular discussions with patients and relatives to ascertain level of satisfaction with ability to continue religious practices.
- Seek views of a random sample of patients by confidential questionnaire following discharge from care.
- Seek views and knowledge of staff by discussion.

Monitoring and Action
- Results of patient satisfaction questionnaires will be recorded and used to inform planning for any change in arrangements.
- Ward manager to initiate discussions for change in overall arrangements for patients to pursue religious practices.

Cross-refs				Data Source(s)	

Figure 4. Use of 'Objectives for Care' in Clinical Audit (NHS Management Executive, 1991).

Background to the first edition

Since its inception, demands upon the Health Service and its employees have increased. Medical technology, demographic change, consumer expectation and managerial concern for improved productivity have all conspired to increase the workload of the caring professions. As demands on the Health Service have intensified there has been a tendency for the individual patient or client's identity and personal needs to become subordinated and obscured. Such observation and criticism have not been restricted to the consumers of the service but have been recognised and acknowledged by the nursing profession.

In an attempt to provide individualised nursing care, the nursing profession in the United Kingdom adopted the 'nursing process' as a broad philosophy for the planning and delivery of nursing care. Definitions of 'nursing process' vary, but common to all is an assumption that professional nursing is a goal-directed, systematic, rational and problem-solving process. The Registered Nurse is accountable for delivery of care based upon an assessment of the individual's needs and subsequent measurement of the effectiveness (evaluation) of the care given. Implementing the nursing process continues to pose significant problems for the profession. The Nurse Education Research Unit's *Report of the Nursing Process Evaluation Working Party* (1986) provides valuable insights into the difficulties being experienced by nurses. In 1983 the North Lincolnshire Health Authority acknowledged that one fundamental obstacle to change was the formal expression of nursing tasks in a 'procedure manual' format. The Chief Nursing Officer recommended that '"guidelines" for nursing practice should be formulated which reflect acceptable standards of nursing care'. It was asserted that 'nursing procedures' were antithetic to an individualised and prescriptive approach to care. Focus on the task inevitably distracted from the individual patient's needs. Additionally the procedure manual restricted professional clinical freedom, and further the inevitable 'DIY Manual' construction of procedures concealed and potentially encouraged disregard for the psychosocial aspects of nursing care. This is not to say that 'procedures' are inaccurate, or that accuracy in performing procedures is not important or necessary. But procedure manuals have tended to dictate specific technical and highly visible nursing actions in a ritualistic manner, leading the nurse through a series of staged instructions towards successful completion of a task. They have not attempted to consider the patient holistically. They generally have no concern for assessment, planning and evaluation of a person's nursing care. Neither do they recognise the role of that person receiving care.

This book is the culmination of four years endeavour by the nurses in one health district, to improve nursing care by expressing its nursing intentions in a manner that shifts the focus from the task to the process, from standard procedures to individual patient needs and from bland ritual to a researched knowledge base.

In developing 'guidelines' for nursing practice, more recently entitled 'objectives for nursing care', the district working party initially examined a variety of nursing models as a foundation for the structure of nursing guidelines. Virginia Henderson's *Basic Principles of Nursing Care* fulfilled the need for a comprehensive and readily understood model for all groups of nurses, midwives and health visitors. Initially, guidelines were received with suspicion, scepticism and even derision. Long-neglected procedure files became trusted, valued and respected—the need for change was challenged. What has been accomplished in preparing this book should not be measured in terms of its completion—the product—but by the quality and rigour of debate that has been necessary for its completion—the process. This debate inevitably has focused on issues of fundamental importance, such as the unique contribution of the nurse, the role of the trained nurse and the student in training, the relationship of nurse and patient and the nurse as the patient's advocate. Consequently *Objectives for Care* is intended to direct nursing intervention in a systematic manner. This book does not dictate specific nursing action but guides the nurse towards the delivery of individual care. It contains suggestions for aspects of care which may be considered, but does not dictate a task which must be completed in a specific way on every occasion.

Expressing objectives for care is a relatively new skill for nurses, and herein resides the utility of this book. More significantly *Objectives for Care* appears to be a useful teaching and learning vehicle for both trained nurses and students. A commonly reported conflict in implementing the nursing process has been the discrepancy between trained nurses' technical skills and students' theoretical knowledge. *Objectives for Care* is a coherent link between theory and practice which is concealed by formally stated 'procedures'. The classification of these objectives remains substantially based upon Henderson's original principles, though these have been expanded and slightly amended by the contributors.

Three additional sections are:

- Helping the patient to express sexuality.
- Helping the patient in pain.
- Helping the dying and bereaved.

However, no specific model for practice is implied. These objectives are proven in a variety of health care settings and can be adapted for use with models using differing assumptions. Each section is supported by a bibliography to encourage and enable nurses to utilise the results of the increasing amount of nursing research in clinical practice. Such research is not merely a useful adjunct. It is frequently asserted that nursing is a 'research-based' profession; more accurately it is a 'much researched' profession. Apposite research must be at the core of nursing practice. Consequently these objectives for care are significantly influenced by nursing research.

It is readily acknowledged that providing personalised health care is not exclusively the responsibility of nurses. It is only possible to deliver high quality care if all participating occupations and professions have shared commitment to its achievement. These objectives, therefore, should be perceived as enabling nurses to contribute to this personalised service, and they contain suggestions about liaison with other providers of health care, including the patient and family.

References

Crow, R. (1981) Research and the standards of nursing care: what is the relationship? *Journal of Advanced Nursing*, **6**, 6, 491–496.

Department of Health (1989a) *Working for Patients*, HMSO, London.

Department of Health (1989b) *Caring for People*, HMSO, London.

Department of Health (1991) *The Patients' Charter*, HMSO, London.

Henderson, V. (1969) *Basic Principles of Nursing Care*, International Council of Nurses, Geneva.

Kitson, A. (1987) Raising standards of clinical practice—the fundamental issue of effective nursing practice, *Journal of Advanced Nursing*, **12**, 321–329.

NHS Management Executive (1991) *Framework of Audit for Nursing Services*.

Nursing Education Research Unit Report 5 (1986) *Report of the Nursing Process Evaluation Working Party*, Kings College, London.

Shaw, C.D. (1980) *Introducing Quality Assurance*, Project Papers 64, London Kings Fund.

Snowley, G.D. and Nicklin, P.J. (1987) *Objectives for Care* (1st Edn), Austen Cornish, London.

Respiration

Introduction
'The healthy individual gives little conscious thought to the activity of breathing. When, for whatever reason, there is some interference with respiratory function, there is need for competent treatment of the cause. The interference may be sudden and traumatic, calling for rapid emergency action and if the difficulty is more than transient, there is a need to support a very anxious, distressed person. The feeling of suffocation and the inability to control such a vital function as breathing can be terrifying.

The person with less sensational breathing difficulty must have equally competent, supportive care because a reduced capacity to breathe can disrupt the function of many other activities of living. If the incapacity is prolonged, this may necessitate a considerable change in life style.'

(Roper, Logan and Tierney: *The Elements of Nursing*)

An adequate supply of oxygen to the tissues requires an efficient cardiovascular system in addition to efficient pulmonary function. Therefore, some people's breathing difficulties may be the result of cardiovascular problems and the objectives include this consideration.

Aims
1. To achieve and maintain for each individual that degree of lung ventilation which is necessary to sustain life and provide the minimum of stress.
2. To provide sufficient education and encouragement to the person for him to be able to avoid future breathing difficulties wherever possible.

Assessment
1. Observe the nature of the person's breathing, skin colour and levels of consciousness.

2. Identify the presence and cause of any anxiety and distress in the person with breathing difficulties.
3. Identify the presence, nature, position and level of any pain associated with breathing.
4. Discuss with the person the nursing help required to achieve the objectives relevant to his condition.

Planning

The plan may involve consideration of one or more of the following:

1. Deciding upon the degree of lung ventilation which is necessary to sustain life but which provides the minimum of stress.
2. The education programme which the person may require in order to avoid future breathing difficulties, wherever possible. (Factors such as smoking, allergies, chest infection and exercise may be considered.)
3. Methods whereby the person may reach maximum independence and avoid the risk of recurrent breathing difficulty.
4. The degree to which privacy and dignity may be maintained, when breathing difficulties threaten these.

Implementation

1. Remove any sudden complete airway obstruction immediately by means of available resources, e.g. fingers, suction, Heimlich manoeuvre, and maintain airway patency by correct positioning or artificial airway.
2. Summon assistance immediately if breathing stops or in cardiac arrest, and commence resuscitation without delay.
3. Remove secretions from the airway to enable oxygen to reach the alveoli. This may necessitate suctioning, chest physiotherapy or help to expectorate sputum.
4. Position the person so that the lungs expand fully and maintain maximum capacity with minimal effort. (This may often be the upright, forward leaning position.)
5. Administer oxygen safely and comfortably as ordered, via mask, nasal catheters, endotracheal tube or oxygen tent and ensure, whenever relevant, that the person understands the therapy and its potential hazards.
6. Ensure adequate humidification of the respiratory tract as ordered to prevent crusting of secretions and to enable their easier removal. This may be achieved by the use of steam inhalations or humidifiers.
7. Administer ordered medications for improvement of lung ventilation, relief of cough or treatment of infection.

8. Provide skilled assistance to persons requiring artificial aids in order to achieve adequate tissue oxygenation, e.g. artificial airway, endotracheal intubation, tracheostomy, underwater seal drainage, ventilator, nebuliser.
9. Introduce and implement appropriate measures for the relief of any anxiety and distress in the person with breathing difficulties.
10. Relieve any pain associated with breathing by the most appropriate means, e.g. through information, touch, local applications, relaxation and medication.
11. Provide health education, e.g. about giving up smoking, the correct use of nebulisers.

Evaluation

Tests for evaluating breathing activity may include the following:

1. Rate and depth of the person's breathing, nature of chest movements, use of accessory muscles for breathing.
2. Peak flow measurement.
3. Skin colour.
4. Presence or absence of confusion.
5. Level of anxiety.
6. Nature and level of any pain.
7. Nature of any cough.
8. Amount and type of sputum produced.
9. Body temperature.
10. Blood pressure.
11. Pulse.
12. Level of the person's understanding about smoking hazards, rehabilitation needs, etc.

Frequency of evaluation will depend on the nature of the care programme, e.g. a patient receiving artificial ventilation will normally require constant observation.

Bibliography
Bagnall, P. and Heslop, A. (1987) Chronic respiratory disease: educating patients at home, *Professional Nurse*, **2**, 9, 293–296.
Blakey, R. (1991) Helping patients not to smoke, *Senior Nurse*, **2**, 2, 18.
Boylan, A. (1985) Respiration: student observations, *Nursing Times*, **81**, 11, 35–38.
McCrissican, D. (1991) Patient education in coronary care, *Nursing Standard*, 26 June, 37.
Miller, J.A. (1989) Blood transfusions: the importance of strict procedures, *Professional Nurse*, **4**, 11, 560–565.
Pritchard, A.P. and David, J. (Eds) (1988) *The Royal Marsden Manual of Clinical Nursing Procedures* (2nd Edn), Harper and Row, London, 71–76,

169–176, 278–284, 361–370

(For details of various research-based cardio-pulmonary procedures).

Roper, N., Logan W.W. and Tierney, A.J. (1990) *The Elements of Nursing* (3rd Edn), Churchill Livingstone, Edinburgh, 136–157.

Speechley, V. and Toovey, J. (1987) Problems in I.V. therapy, *Professional Nurse*, **2**, 8, 240–242.

Eating and drinking

Introduction

Whilst eating and drinking are normally highly pleasurable activities, their basic purpose is to provide the nutrients necessary for body growth and to maintain adequate body function and repair. Mealtimes can also be important social events, where ritual, culture and major life events may be celebrated.

Attitudes to food may be influenced from infancy by the nature of the baby's experience with feeding, and by customs related to culture and religion. Eating independently and choosing what and when we eat are activities exercised by us all from a very early age. Interference with these activities, for whatever reason, may result in some degree of malnutrition or body fluid disturbance which may even become life-threatening.

> 'If the nurse is an intelligent being and not a mere carrier of diets to and from the patient, let her exercise her intelligence in these things.'
> (Florence Nightingale, 1860)

Aims

1. To ensure the correct nutrition and hydration of each individual, based on a secure knowledge of recommended daily intakes of nutrients and fluid.
2. To prevent avoidable malnutrition by providing appropriate education to individuals and their families.

Assessment

1. Assess the understanding by individuals and their families of the general principles of nutrition and the contribution of healthy eating towards positive health.

2. Ascertain the person's build, body weight and skin condition and observe for signs of poor nutrition and dehydration.
3. Discuss, with the person if possible, the need for special diet as part of his medical treatment, e.g. for diabetes mellitus, renal disease, obesity.
4. Identify the person's normal eating and drinking habits, including timing of meals and associated patterns of hygiene, so that there may be as little disruption as possible.
5. Be aware of any pain and distressing treatments, nausea, anxiety, depression or poor appetite which may interfere with normal eating and drinking and its enjoyment.
6. Observe for any psychological disturbance which may produce or be the result of extremes of eating and drinking habit, e.g. anorexia nervosa, alcoholism.
7. Identify any physical handicap or positional difficulty which may interfere with a person's independence in eating and drinking.
8. Observe the condition of the mouth, gums, tongue, teeth or dentures of the person, in case of underlying causes of chewing and swallowing difficulties.
9. Observe for signs of oedema and dehydration.
10. Discuss any cultural or religious customs which may affect a person's eating and drinking.
11. Check the particular weaning programme of an infant as indicated by accurate assessment with the parents, and assess the parents' abilities to cope with infant feeding demands.

Planning

The plan may involve consideration of one or more of the following:

1. A programme of co-operation with colleagues in other disciplines to provide a programme of support, education and advice to patients and their families about the contribution of healthy eating towards good health.
2. The education and support programme which will be required by those people who require help in overcoming specific difficulties in eating and drinking, e.g. where special diets form part of their treatment, those suffering the effect of alcohol or food abuse, those requiring advice on dental hygiene and treatment, mealtime training programmes for people with learning disability.
3. The required flexibility of timing of meals and sufficient time for each person to take food and drink at their own pace.
4. The need for organising possible relief of pain, timing of therapy, and positioning of the person so that meals may be fully enjoyed.
5. Any necessary measures for the relief of nausea and poor appetite.

These may include comfort and support, avoidance of certain foods, anti-emetic drugs as prescribed, tempting snacks from home, ice cubes to suck, and involving the person in food choice.

6. The use of appropriate utensils and physical help to enable a disabled person to strive for independence in eating and drinking.

7. Requirements for instructing the mothers of new-born infants on the principles of infant feeding, e.g. practical advice on breast feeding and artificial feeding.

8. Continuance of weaning programmes for infants and provision of feeds most appropriate for young children.

9. The special needs of the person requiring artificial feeding or hydration, to ensure that a balanced diet and fluid intake is given in complete safety, e.g. nasogastric, gastrostomy, total parenteral nutrition, intravenous therapy. This may involve liaison with the dietician, and with catering, medical and pharmacy staff.

10. Adequate and accurate preparation for people who require a period of fasting prior to surgery or clinical investigations.

11. Provision of an eating and drinking pattern which will meet a person's religious or cultural customs.

12. Special provisions for children in hospital, whose separation from family and home may produce regressive feeding behaviour patterns. Full parental involvement would be a consideration here.

13. Requirements for training or retraining in the selection and purchase of food, according to the age and ability of the person, e.g. rehabilitation in mental health, preparation for independence for a person with learning disability.

Implementation

1. Provide the most appropriate social and physical environment in which people, of whatever age, may enjoy the social activity of eating and drinking.

2. Work in co-operation with other hospital and community services to provide a varied choice of meals.

3. Explain to the person the procedure for ordering and choosing meals and ensure that appropriate selection of food occurs, especially where the person is unable to manage this independently, e.g. children, elderly people.

4. Provide gracious and dextrous assistance to those people who are unable to feed themselves, so that their dignity and comfort are fully maintained.

5. Provide adequate facilities to people before and after meals so

that their normal standards of mouth and hand hygiene are
maintained as desired.

6. Provide suitable protection (clothing, napkins) to those people
who require special help during mealtimes.
7. Inform and support the person who requires advice about
healthy eating towards good health.
8. Ensure cleanliness and safety in all food handlers.

Evaluation

1. The person's level of satisfaction with quantity and quality of
food and drink taken, and time of serving meals.
2. Presence or absence of dyspepsia, flatulence, nausea, pain and/or
other discomforts associated with eating and drinking.
3. Body weight.
4. General physical appearance.
5. The nature of skin and mucous membranes for signs of dehydration.
6. Presence or absence of oedema.
7. Record of person's fluid intake and output.
8. Presence or absence of abnormalities in urine.
9. Nature of faeces where abnormalities may be suspected.
10. Level of understanding and knowledge about diet.

Bibliography

Barnes, K.E. (1990) An examination of nurses' feelings about patients with
specific feeding needs, *Journal of Advanced Nursing*, June, 703.
(Excellent research report about the views of patients and nurses about
meeting feeding needs, which has implications for nursing practice in this
area).
Bockus, S. (1991) Trouble shooting your tube feedings, *American Journal of
Nursing*, May, 24.
(Solutions for all major tube feeding dilemmas, followed by a multiple-
choice test).
British Dietetic Association (1988) *Manual of Dietetic Practice*, Blackwell,
Oxford.
Brown, K. (1991) Improving intakes, *Nursing Times*, 15 May, 64.
(Provides plans for making hospital patients' diets more adequate).
Carter, A. and Bell, S. (1988) *Food in Focus*, John Wiley and Sons Inc., New
York.
Hamilton-Smith, S. (1981) *Nil by Mouth*, Royal College of Nursing, London.
Holmes, S. (1991) Planning for the best start in life: a guide to infant feeding,
Professional Nurse, **6**, 4, 200–205.
Jones, D.C. (1977) *Food for Thought*, Royal College of Nursing, London.
Michell, C. (1987) Steadying the hand that feeds, *Journal of Nursing*, March,
293–296.
Pearson, M. (1990) Small steps to progress, *Nursing Times*, 17 October, 28.
(Using Peplau's nursing model to help a person with an alcohol problem).

Roper, N., Logan, W.W. and Tierney, A.J. (1990) *The Elements of Nursing* (3rd Edn), Churchill Livingstone, Edinburgh, pp 158–182.

Elimination

Introduction

Elimination is an activity which all individuals perform regularly throughout life. It includes micturition, defaecation, expiration and perspiration, whereby the body is rid of metabolic waste products and unabsorbed food residue.

A person responds to the need to eliminate wherever he is, whatever he is doing and whatever the time of day. A most important characteristic of defaecation and micturition is that they are normally performed in private, though social and cultural differences can affect this pattern. This section is concerned, particularly, with these two functions.

Aims

1. Wherever possible, to achieve and maintain a pattern of elimination as close as possible to each person's normal pattern.
2. To provide the necessary support and aids when the normal pattern of elimination will never be regained.
3. To provide education and encouragement to prevent future problems arising.

Assessment

1. Discuss with the person the help required to establish normal frequency of elimination.
2. Establish what vocabulary the person uses and understands regarding the process of elimination.
3. Establish what is a normal frequency of elimination for the individual and check any changes in this by observation.
4. Determine the nature and pattern of any incontinence.
5. Identify the level and nature of any pain associated with elimination.

6. Discuss with or observe in the person any abnormalities in the act of elimination, or in its products.
7. Identify what the person needs to learn to overcome the problems of elimination with reference to diet, appliances, behaviour, habits and personal hygiene.

Planning

The plan may involve consideration of one or more of the following:

1. A programme which achieves a pattern of elimination which is acceptable to the individual patient and, where appropriate, the family.
2. An interdisciplinary education programme for the individual and family to improve knowledge and outcomes of elimination activities.
3. Counselling when abnormalities of elimination cause emotional distress.
4. Management of physical discomforts, e.g. pain and soreness resulting from incontinence, constipation, the presence of a stoma.
5. The use of appropriate aids and appliances, to ensure satisfactory elimination.
6. Provision of accurate information about a suitable range of methods and resources which may be used to overcome a person's elimination problems, e.g. their suitability for the home environment and the person's pattern of life.

Implementation

1. Ensure that the individual's privacy and dignity are maintained.
2. Relieve any pain associated with elimination by the most appropriate means.
3. Prevent cross infection by ensuring safe disposal of excreta.
4. Protect the surrounding areas of skin when faecal or urinary incontinence is present.
5. Prevent and treat faecal impaction and constipation.
6. Provide skilled assistance to people with colostomies, ileostomies or ileal conduit or other medical intervention to ensure they have sufficient support and knowledge on the care of their stomas, catheters, and surrounding skin.
7. Provide adequate care for people with indwelling catheters to prevent infection.
8. Administer rectal suppositories and enemata when prescribed, e.g. for bowel preparation prior to operative procedures.

9. Provide facilities for personal hygiene after elimination.
10. Adjust dietary intake, as necessary, to maintain satisfactory bowel and bladder action.
11. Use psychological and physical methods to relax tense abdominal muscles as necessary, e.g. warmth to the lower abdomen, relaxation programmes.

Evaluation

The following may be used in evaluating this activity:

1. Person's level of satisfaction with the privacy and dignity available to him.
2. Person's level of satisfaction with the frequency and ease of elimination.
3. The person's expressions, overt or covert, of self-esteem.
4. Expressions of pain or discomfort, by the patient, associated with the process of elimination or the need to eliminate.
5. Observation of the skin for any rashes or soreness.
6. The level of satisfaction expressed by the person or family, with the use of aids and appliances.
7. Monitoring the progress of the person towards independence in elimination or, when this is not realistic, the satisfaction of the individual or family in the management of the problem.
8. Observations for changes in the frequency and amount of elimination and its products, e.g. colour and consistency of urine and faeces.
9. Level of knowledge and understanding of the person who requires long-term or permanent changes of elimination habit, e.g. the person with colostomy, ileostomy, indwelling catheter, intermittent self-catheterisation, continual ambulatory peritoneal dialysis.

Bibliography

Barrett, J. (1990) Treating faecal incontinence, *Nursing Times*, August 15th, 66.

Brown, J., Meikle, J. and Webb, C. (1991) Collecting midstream specimens of urine (MSSU)—The Research Base, *Nursing Times*, March 27th, 49–52. (Study of medical and nursing articles about MSSU collection, between 1956 and 1989: raises important questions about the validity of instructions for collecting these specimens).

Burgener, S. (1987) Justification of closed intermittent urinary catheter irrigation/instillation: a review of current research and practice, *Journal of Advanced Nursing*, **12**, 2, 229–233.

Hughes, A. (1991) Life with a stoma, *Nursing Times*, 19th June, 67–68. (How patients try to come to terms with their new body image).

Milne, B., Joachim, G. and Niedhart, J. (1986) A stress management programme for inflammatory bowel disease patients, *Journal of Advanced Nursing*, **11**, 5, 566.

Roper, N., Logan, W.W. and Tierney, A.J. (1990) *The Elements of Nursing* (3rd Edn), Churchill Livingstone, Edinburgh, 183–204.

Tierney, A. (1973) Toilet training, *Nursing Times*, **69**, 1140–1145.

Southern, D. and Henderson, P. (1990) Tackling incontinence, *Nursing Times*, March 7th, 36.

(How toileting practices with elderly patients were improved).

Thomas, B. (1991) Nurses' prescription of stoma appliances, *Nursing Standard*, 16th January, 25.

(Information about the role of the stoma nurse).

Wheeler, V. (1990) A new kind of loving, *Professional Nurse*, **5**, 9, 492–496.

(Effect of continence problems on sexuality).

Wilson, J. and Roe, B. (1986) Nursing management of patients with indwelling urethral catheter, *Clinical Nursing Practice*, **14**, 76–100.

Mobility

Introduction

The ability to move the body freely is one of the valued activities of living. The loss of ability to move any part of the body is one of the major tragedies that can happen to a person. Whether loss of movement is transient or permanent, it can lead to particular problems, e.g. pressure sores, deep vein thrombosis, muscle wastage, joint degeneration. It is therefore important to do everything possible to prevent degeneration and the complications of immobility and to hasten recovery and restoration of movement.

Aims

1. To achieve and maintain, for each individual, the maximum possible degree of mobilisation.
2. To provide social and psychological comfort when there is interference with mobility which results in loss of freedom.
3. To increase peoples' awareness in the importance of mobility and the principles relevant to programmes of exercise.

Assessment

1. Observe, and discuss with the person, the present level of mobility.
2. Identify the type and extent of any mobility difficulties. This may require involvement from other experts in the health care team, e.g. physiotherapists.
3. Observe for and discuss any pain, and its degree, in relation to the person's mobility difficulties.
4. Assess the skin for abnormal signs, e.g. discolouration, sores, loss of sensation.
5. Assess the person's risk for the development of pressure sores.

6. Measure skin pressures on vulnerable body surfaces for any person likely to have long periods of immobility for whatever reason (e.g. lengthy surgical operations, following stroke and other neurological trauma, unconsciousness).
7. Identify any present or future requirements for therapeutic immobilisation, e.g. with orthopaedic patients, those requiring major surgery.
8. Assess the use of physical aids and other resources and benefits to support maximum mobility.
9. Assess the degree to which restricted mobility is affecting the psychological and social status of the person.

Planning

The plan may involve consideration of one or more of the following:

1. Ensuring the person's dignity and privacy are maintained at all times.
2. A programme of co-operation with other disciplines to improve and maintain mobility to the maximum level possible.
3. Methods employed to improve the person's motivation, responsibility and acceptance of planned exercise programmes.
4. The necessary education and support to the relatives, or other carers, who will assume major responsibility for continuing care, e.g. with the stroke patient.
5. Elimination of pain and discomfort associated with mobilisation.
6. The use of physical aids and equipment to enable the fullest possible degree of mobility and prevention of the complications of immobility.
7. A clear programme for prevention of pressure sores, and for treatment of developed sores.
8. Prevention of undue exhaustion for the person.
9. Improving knowledge, understanding and acceptance of the benefits of exercise towards optimum health and well being.
10. Information for the person and relatives about social, financial and voluntary benefits available in helping to overcome mobility difficulties.

Implementation

1. Provide support, empathy and encouragement to help the person to face the problems of sudden or gradual immobility difficulties (e.g. rheumatoid arthritis).
2. Ensure the person is given and takes as much responsibility as possible in all activities of living.

3. Carry out with, or for, the person, isotonic, isometric and passive exercises as required.
4. Use relevant pressure-relieving surfaces, and other aids where necessary, in the management of people at risk of developing pressure sores.
5. Collaborate with medical and physiotherapy staff in carrying out mobility programmes with individuals.
6. Provide properly measured and fitted mobility aids wherever appropriate and ensure that the person is taught how to use them effectively, e.g. wheelchairs, crutches, other walking aids.
7. Arrange for the involvement of other services in preparation for continuing improvement and maintenance of mobility, e.g. Community Care personnel, local authority services.
8. Lift safely at all times, in order to maintain personal health and mobility.

Evaluation

In the evaluating strategy the following factors should be considered:

1. Levels of motor ability and stamina to complete exercise programmes.
2. The person's mental state.
3. The effects of immobility and the care programme on relatives or other carers.
4. Levels of pain.
5. The condition of the skin and progress of healing of any pressure sores.
6. The person's knowledge and use of relevant mechanical aids.
7. Levels of independence.

Bibliography

Chapman, E.J. and Chapman, R. (1986) Treatment of pressure sores: the state of the art, *Clinical Nursing Practice*, **14**, 105–124.

Clark, M. (1991) Comparison of the pressure redistributing attributes of a selection of bed mattresses used to prevent pressure sores, *Journal of Tissue Viability*, July, 65–67.

Davies, K., Strickland, J., Lawrence, V., Duncan, A. and Rome, J. (1991) The hidden mortality from pressure sores, *Journal of Tissue Viability*, January, 18. (Article based on research which suggests that mortality related to pressure sores is under reported and may go unrecognised).

Dealey, C. (1990) How are you supporting your patients? *Professional Nurse* **6**, 3, 134–141.
(Review of pressure relieving equipment).

Dealey, C, Earwacker, T. and Eden, L. (1991) Are your patients sitting comfortably? *Journal of Tissue Viability*, April, 36–39.
(Evaluation of a new armchair showing improvement in pressure relief and improved posture as well as a positive response from the patients involved).

Dobson, M. (1991) Back pain prevention: collaborative techniques in the workplace, *Health Education Journal*, **50**, 2, 91.

Gould, D. (1986) Pressure sore prevention and treatment: an example of nurses' failure to implement research findings, *Journal of Advanced Nursing*, **11**, 4, 389–394.

Herbert, R. (1991) A patient's view, *Journal of Tissue Viability*, April.

(Thought provoking article about the best pressure relieving surface for a 25-year-old man with spina bifida and a large pressure sore on his buttocks).

Judd, M. (1989) *Mobility: Patient Problems and Nursing Care*, Heinmann Nursing, Oxford.

(Excellent book, with invaluable guidance about helping people with mobility problems from the very young to the very old, and for a wide range of health care settings).

McCall, J. (1991) Watch your back, *Nursing Standard*, 6 March, 50.

(Health and safety article about the need for nurses to protect their backs by caring as much for their own safety as they do for their patients).

Norton, D., McLaren, R. and Exton-Smith, A.N. (1975) *An Investigation of Geriatric Nursing Problems in Hospital*, Churchill Livingstone, Edinburgh.

Waterlow, J. (1991) The Waterlow pressure sore prevention/treatment policy, *Professional Nurse*, **6**, 5, 258–264.

(The Waterlow card has been a valuable tool in the assessment and prevention of pressure sores. Its use not only protect patients from unnecessary sores but also health authorities from legal action).

Note The *Journal of Tissue Viability*, published quarterly, is an unrivalled source of research abstracts about skin care and pressure relief.

Communication

Introduction
Communication is fundamental to the work of the nurse. To be an effective communicator is to assist people in many aspects of their daily living. To communicate is to 'impart', 'transmit', 'receive' or 'share'. It is extremely difficult for the carer not to convey personal ideas, opinions, feelings, bias and prejudice although, sometimes, it is useful to share these. Communication is fraught with good intentions and real difficulties.

The two-way process of communication is not restricted to the use of language. It cannot be assumed that effective communication has taken place because words have been exchanged. Effective communication occurs only when all participants have a shared understanding of what has been communicated.

Aim
To promote effective communication enabling expression of needs and feelings, in order to plan and give individual care.

Assessment
1. Be aware of different cultural practices in the art of communication.
2. Assess the person's moods and appreciate the influence this has on communication, e.g. nervousness, depression, aggression.
3. Establish the person's ability to understand and, therefore, respond to information and instructions.
4. Assess language difficulties, differences in dialect and pronunciation, children's special use of words.
5. Establish the person's ability to read or write.
6. Establish the person's level of sensory functions, as any loss may affect ability to receive information.

7. Assess the presence of any physical or psychological pain which may be a potential barrier to communication.
8. Assess the effects of drugs (prescribed or unprescribed). Certain drugs affect the person's level of consciousness, resulting in communication breakdown, e.g. drowsiness, excitement, dryness of mouth.

Planning

The plan may involve consideration of one or more of the following:

1. Arrangements needed to provide an environment which is conducive to communication, e.g. it is warm, quiet, soothing, private.
2. Planned intervention to reduce barriers of communication, e.g. help of an interpreter, joint planning with speech therapist, removal of formalities, referral to remedial agencies for illiteracy.
3. Requirements to involve all members of the health care team in the process of communication.
4. Use of special physical aids as necessary, e.g. glasses, hearing aids, picture cards.
5. Appropriate education programme for the individual and family to improve and maintain satisfactory levels of communication.
6. Special therapeutic programmes, in consultation with specialists, e.g. reminiscence therapy, drama, art, psychotherapy.

Implementation

1. Provide a relaxed atmosphere for the person to communicate freely.
2. Employ different means of communication, in addition to speech, e.g. facial expression, gestures, eye contact, writing and pictures.
3. When consistent with the individual's preferred style of communication, use touch to convey concern and provide comfort.
4. Obtain the person's consent for referral to remedial agencies, if such help is considered appropriate.
5. Translate technical language and avoid jargon to increase comprehension and reduce apprehension.
6. With the person's consent, provide accurate verbal and written communication on the individual's condition and progress to specified relatives, friends and other health care workers.
7. Promote in all health care workers the need for constant

observation of the person's speech patterns, tone of voice, eye contact, body space requirements, language and sensory impairments. These can give some indications of the person's mental state.

Evaluation

To evaluate the effectiveness of communication the following points should be noted:

1. The physical and mental state of the person.
2. The person's level of understanding of information, materials and aids used, reading and writing ability.
3. The person's level of sensory perception.
4. Verbal and non-verbal expressions of the individual.
5. Information from interpreters, remedial teachers, speech therapists, family and friends.
6. Effects of any drugs on the person's comunication ability.
7. Success or failure of any aids used.
8. Information from all health care team members.

Bibliography

Burnard, P. (1990) *Learning Human Skills* (2nd Edn), Butterworth Heinmann Ltd, Oxford.

Ingram, R. (1991) Learning difficulties and communication, *Nursing Standard*, 24 April, 36–39.
(Special communication needs and problems of people with learning disability and the need for attitude changes on a large scale).

Jolly, J. (1986) Communicating with children, *Professional Nurse*, **1**, 10, 266–267.

Kagan, C. (Ed) (1985) *Interpersonal Skills in Nursing*, Croom Helm Ltd, Kent.

Munday, A. (1973) *Physiological Measures of Anxiety in Hospital Patients*, Royal College of Nursing, London.

Porritt, L. (1984) *Communication: Choices for Nurses*, Longman, Singapore, pp 48–61.

Home, E. (Ed) (1992) *Effective Communication* (2nd Edn), Wolfe Publishing.
(Compilation of articles first published in the *Professional Nurse* magazine: covers a wide range of difficult situations in which nurses need special communication skills).

Rogers, C. (1967) *On Becoming a Person* (2nd Edn), Constable, London.

Roper, N., Logan, W.W. and Tierney, A.J. (1990) *The Elements of Nursing* (3rd Edn), Churchill Livingstone, Edinburgh, pp 108–135.

Swan, I. and Tolson, D. (1991) 'Facing up to deafness' and 'Gentle persuasion', *Nursing Times*, 5 June, 26–31.
(Breaking down barriers to communication and helping people come to terms with deafness).

Wilkinson, S. (1991) Factors which influence how nurses communicate with cancer patients, *Journal of Advanced Nursing*, June, 677–688.
(Research which shows that effective communication does not just depend on the acquisition of the skills required to communicate).

Wilson-Barnett, J. (1986) Reducing stress in hospital, *Clinical Nursing Practice*, **14**.

Dressing and undressing

Introduction
People wear clothes to keep warm, to express cultural or religious differences, to inform society of status, group membership or professional identity, or for actual physical protection. The importance, to some people, of clothes and personal appearance, is reflected in the amount of time and money which may be spent in achieving the desired image. Deprivation of the usual pattern of dressing and attention to appearance may have a profound effect on an individual.

Aims
1. To ensure that each individual wears clothing which provides comfort and dignity at all times.
2. To provide facilities and aids for people to adopt a dressing and undressing programme which leaves them feeling physically and mentally at ease at all times.

Assessment
1. Ascertain the person's cultural, religious and fashion aspects of clothing.
2. Ascertain the differences between day and night attire, if any, for the person (in some cultures, the same clothing is worn during the day and night).
3. Check for any incontinence or other problems which may require the use of special clothing.
4. Discuss with the individual their likes and dislikes and needs in the matter of clothing, e.g. colour, style and fit.
5. Identify any difficulties with fastenings to garments, and assess their suitability to the needs of the individual.
6. Identify any infestation of clothing, if present.

7. Assess the suitability of clothing for existing climatic conditions.

Planning

The plan may involve consideration of one or more of the following:

1. Methods of promoting maximum independence by training or retraining the individual and relatives in the skills of dressing and undressing. (Other health care professionals may be involved in such a programme.)
2. Provision of encouragement and motivation to the person to dress and undress, e.g. rehabilitation programme for the disabled or apathetic person, special occasions to stimulate interest.
3. Preparations and referrals which may be necessary to obtain specially designed clothes or shoes for the person whose disability suggests that these may be helpful.
4. Identification of any necessary pain relief.
5. Special measures which may be required to prevent discomfort and skin damage, e.g. avoid restrictive clothing and allergenic fabric.
6. Information and education to the person and relatives about prevention of overheating or underheating of the body, e.g. mother and infant, the elderly.
7. Special measures required for training or retraining in the correct selection, purchase and care of clothing, depending on the age and ability of the person, e.g. rehabilitation in mental health, promoting independence for the person with learning disability.
8. Teaching of grooming, where necessary.

Implementation

1. Provide privacy and a safe environment for dressing and undressing.
2. Encourage full expression of cultural, religious and fashion aspects of clothing for all individuals.
3. Ensure the use of individual personal clothing and ensure that each person has a sufficient supply for changing whenever necessary.
4. Provide aids, as necessary, and train people in their full use to assist in dressing and undressing.
5. Provide suitable laundry and storage facilities for the individual's clothes.
6. Safeguard all personal clothing against theft, loss or incorrect laundering.

7. Obtain protective clothing for individuals as necessary, e.g. napkins or protective clothing for mealtimes, anti-embolism stockings, fire-retardant materials.
8. Use correct methods in managing infested clothing, to protect others from infestation.
9. Ensure a dignified appearance and comfort for an individual who leaves the ward for transfer or to await investigative procedures in other departments.
10. Consult with members of the clothing industry about the needs and desires of individuals for a smart and fashionable appearance, despite a physical or psychological disability.

Evaluation

One or more of the following may be involved in evaluating dressing and undressing:

1. Person's level of satisfaction with appearance and general physical comfort of clothing.
2. Observation to ensure a neat and dignified appearance for the individual.
3. Observation of the skin for any rashes or lesions which may be caused by unsuitable clothing.
4. Expressions of pain or discomfort by the person, which may be preventing the full activity of dressing and undressing.
5. Adequacy of specially designed clothing or footwear, e.g. its size, shape, acceptance by the person.

Bibliography

Adams, S. (1987) The relationship of clothing to self esteem in elderly patients, *Nursing Times*, 9 September, 42–45.

Clements, S. (1987) Aids to disabled living, *Nursing Times*, 17 June, 54.

Davidson, L. (1989) Time for a change, *Nursing Times*, 29 November, 26–29. (Patients wearing their own clothes).

Hurst, K. and Ward, L. (1991) Modesty in ICUs—suitable clothing for patients in ICUs, *Nursing Times*, 10 July, 40.

Mitchell, S.C.M. (1991) Everyday aids and appliances: dressing aids, *British Medical Journal*, 19 January, 167–169.

Roper, N., Logan, W.W. and Tierney, A.J. (1990) *The Elements of Nursing* (3rd Edn), Churchill Livingstone, Edinburgh, pp 205–232.

Trevelyan, J. (1988) Dress code, *Nursing Times*, 23 November, 21. (Provision of clothing to long stay patients).

Body temperature

Introduction

Body temperature is determined by the balance between *heat production* and *heat loss*. If they are exactly equal the body temperature neither rises nor falls. Regulatory systems in the body are always at work to keep heat production and heat loss approximately equal thereby maintaining a normal body temperature.

Man is able to adapt to changes in environmental temperature so that his scope of activity is broad. From childhood we learn to adapt clothing, heating and ventilation to meet our needs. In adulthood the budgeting of finances to cover heating costs is an additional responsibility. Controlling body temperature is an important activity of living and is carried out, consciously and unconsciously, as part of man's existence.

Body temperature records can provide vital information about a person's progress during a programme of health care. Its recording should be timely and accurate.

Aims

1. To achieve and maintain the individual's normal body temperature, irrespective of the temperature of the environment, thus freeing the person from discomfort.
2. To provide adequate education so that individuals are aware of the dangers of abnormally high or low body temperatures and are able to maintain a normal body temperature.

Assessment

1. Measure body temperature using the most appropriate method, according to the general state of the person, e.g. level of consciousness, age, mental state, pain.

2. Observe for other physical signs of abnormal temperature, e.g. feel and colour of the skin, lethargy/unconsciousness, condition of extremities, convulsions in infants.
3. Identify needs or problems which may affect body temperature adversely, e.g. living conditions, degree of mobility, mental state, presence of infection.
4. Assess the person's knowledge, initiative and skill to dress appropriately or adjust room temperature in accordance with climatic conditions.

Planning

The plan may involve consideration of one or more of the following:

1. Defining suitable activities to generate body heat. (This is particularly relevant for those who are sedentary.)
2. Education and training plans for those who are not fully competent in maintaining their own body temperature.
3. Information and advice to relatives and other carers about the effects of extremes of environment or body temperature on the very young and the very old.
4. Information about effective clothing, controlling environmental temperatures at home, and help available from other agencies, in order to maintain normal body temperature.
5. Methods whereby normal body temperature may be restored safely, e.g. slow warming in hypothermia, tepid sponging and air cooling in pyrexia.

Implementation

1. Promote the individual's privacy, dignity and individuality when taking appropriate action in maintaining/controlling their body temperature.
2. Avoid rapid rewarming and application of direct heat to the person with hypothermia (peripheral vasodilatation and circulatory collapse may result).
3. Administer conservative treatment for controlling raised body temperature, e.g. tepid sponging when necessary, cool the environment.
4. Maintain adequate fluid and food intake to prevent further complications of dehydration and increased metabolic rate in the pyrexic person.
5. Summon intervention when an extreme rise or fall of an individual's body temperature has been identified.
6. Collect any relevant specimen which may help in the diagnosis

of the possible causes of changes in body temperature, e.g. specimens from the respiratory and urinary tracts, to check for infection.

7. Administer prescribed treatment for controlling the cause of the rise or fall in body temperature, e.g. specific infection, thyroid disorder.

Evaluation

This should be a continuous process and its timing will depend on the needs of the person and may include the following:

1. Nursing observation of changes in the individual's body temperature.
2. The person's level of comfort concerning his body temperature.

For a person with irregularities in body temperature, evaluation may also include regular monitoring of the following:

3. Level of pulse rate, respiration rate and blood pressure.
4. Intake and output of food/drink.
5. Mental state of person.
6. Physical state of person.
7. Skin condition.
8. Person's awareness of the problem.

Bibliography

Brown, S. (1990) Temperature taking: getting it right, *Nursing Standard Supplement*, 12 December.

DHSS (1972) *Keeping Warm in Winter*.
   (Simple guidance notes for elderly people and their carers).

Goodall, C. (1986) Heat trials: testing the accuracy of thermometer readings, *Nursing Times*, 19 February, 46.

Hillman, H. (1987) The cold that kills, *Nursing Times*, **83**, 4, 19–20.

Nichols, G.A. and Kucha, D.H. (1972) Taking adult temperatures: oral measurements, *American Journal of Nursing*, **72**, 1091–1092.

Roper, N., Logan, W.W. and Tierney, A.J. (1990) *The Elements of Nursing* (3rd Edn) Churchill Livingstone, Edinburgh, pp.238–245.

Wright, J. (1991) Accidental hypothermia, *Professional Nurse*, **6**, 4, 197–199.

Personal hygiene

Introduction

Good personal hygiene usually refers to those measures taken to keep skin, hair, nails and mouth clean and in good condition. These activities may also provide comfort and relaxation, stimulation of the circulation, freedom from infection, and improved self-esteem through improved appearance and a feeling of well being.

Illness, both physical and psychological, can lead to acute alterations of a person's normal standard of hygiene. Change of environment, loss of independence, unfamiliar routines and lack of privacy may all contribute to major interference with these personal and important activities. Enforced change in the normal processes of cleanliness may mean that a person has to learn to cope with changes or be helped to achieve agreeable standards of hygiene under difficult circumstances. Whatever these circumstances may be, it is important that rigid routines are avoided if self-image, self-esteem and positive attitudes for the person are to be maintained.

Aims

1. To promote hygiene and comfort for the person receiving health care.
2. To improve and maintain a person's independence in hygiene activities, whenever appropriate.
3. To provide adequate information and support to the person who requires education in matters of hygiene.

Assessment

1. Establish the person's normal routine for hygiene, including cultural or religious practices which are important to the individual.

2. Assess the effect of the person's usual environment upon the ability to stay clean, e.g. basic facilities may be lacking.
3. Assess the factors that impair the person's personal hygiene, e.g. physical disability, anything which reduces independence.
4. Identify the most likely to be affected by self-neglect if left unattended, i.e. the very young, the confused, the unmotivated, the homeless, the lonely and those lacking the necessary basic skills.
5. Assess the influence of pain, discomfort and distressing treatments which interfere with a person's normal desires for cleanliness.
6. Check for signs of skin disease, injury or infestation.
7. Identify any special requirements in cleansing, e.g. for the person with a stoma or urethral catheter.

Planning

The plan may involve consideration of one or more of the following:

1. A programme of hygiene which allows the person to maintain their normal pattern and independence, wherever this is compatible with their total health care needs.
2. Means of providing assistance to the person who is not fully independent in maintaining good hygiene, including the provision of appropriate physical aids or support from other personnel, e.g. occupational therapist, hairdresser, chiropodist.
3. Planned treatment for any skin or hair infestation which may be present.
4. Any necessary education and training to promote independence.
5. Consideration of the need for special nutrition or hydration to improve skin care.
6. Investigations, wherever appropriate, of home circumstances for good hygiene.
7. Checking for any allergic response to soaps, lotions etc.

Implementation

1. Maintain the person's privacy, dignity and individuality during all hygiene activities.
2. Respect the individual's preference for methods and timing of hygiene activities.
3. Provide, or make the necessary arrangements for provision at home, those necessary appliances to enable a person to improve independence and safety in maintaining hygiene, e.g. non-slip mats, special flannels, toothbrushes, combs, required bathroom

alterations. (The help and advice of the National Disabled Living Foundation or other professionals may be required.)

4. Avoid the use of irritant soaps, lotions, shampoos, etc., if the person has a particular sensitivity to these.
5. Avoid undue fatigue to the person who requires major intervention in maintaining hygiene.
6. Instruct the patient and family in the importance of adequate hygiene, if necessary.
7. Observe the skin around bony prominences, sensitive areas and areas subject to pressure, for signs of damage or inflammation.
8. Provide help and advice to parents of new-born infants, to improve and maintain confidence in bathing their babies.
9. Ensure safety from physical injury or cross infection during hygiene activities.

Evaluation
The following factors may be considered:

1. The level of the person's satisfaction with personal hygiene.
2. The ability of the person to manage aids and the level of understanding about their use.
3. The condition of the skin, hair, mouth, teeth and nails.
4. The presence or absence of abrasions, sores, physical injury.
5. The effects of treatments for infestation.
6. The person's general physical and mental state.
7. Specific progress in training or rehabilitation programmes for hygiene activities.

Bibliography
Cluroe, S. (1990) How to deal with head lice, *Nursing*, 9 August, 24.
Pearson, A. (1987) *Living in a Plaster Cast*, Royal College of Nursing, London, pp 80–82.
Roper, N., Logan, W.W. and Tierney, A. (1990) *Elements of Nursing* (3rd Edn), Churchill Livingstone, Edinburgh, pp 205–232.
Thompson, J. (1990) Oral hygiene and dental care, *Community Outlook*, January, 10.
(Importance of dental health as part of general nursing care: covers oral hygiene for young and old).
Trentor-Roth, P. and Creason, N. (1986) Nurse-administered oral hygiene: is there a scientific basis? *Journal of Advanced Nursing*, **11**, 3, 323–331.
Webster, R., Thompson, D., Bowman, G. and Sutton, T. (1988) Patients and nurses' opinions about bathing, *Nursing Times* (Occasional Paper), 14 September, 54.
(This research paper describes how nurses and patients often have rather discordant views about bathing and what is important: recommended reading for appreciation of the need for individualised care in bathing and other matters).

Wells, R. and Trostle, K. (1984) Creative hairwashing techniques for immobilized patients, *Nursing*, **14**, 1, 47–51.

Wilson, M. (1987) *Occupational Therapy in Long Term Psychiatry* (2nd Edn), Churchill Livingstone, Edinburgh.
(Commonsense approach to care planning and implementation of social skills training for both the mentally ill and people with learning disability).

Wright, L. (1990) Bathing by towel, *Nursing Times*, 24 January, 36.
(Description of an alternative to the ritual bed bath, that has saving both in time and money).

Safety

Introduction

Environmental awareness begins shortly after birth and continues throughout life, allowing people choice in their personal environment. This is true even for the disabled who devote energy towards accomplishing tasks to fulfil the wish of being master of their personal environment.

The health and quality of our lives are greatly affected by the influence of the environment. As A.H. Maslow (1943) suggested, we all have a safety and self-preservation need, which we endeavour to meet while mastering the environment.

Promoting a safe environment is one of the many functions of the nurse. The environment can be influenced by many events, including industrial and technological growth, infection and violence. The promotion of a safe environment, including that of the hospital, makes good economic sense as well as improving and maintaining the nation's health.

Aims

1. To help detect ill effects of the environment on health and the ill effects of people's actions on the environment.
2. To improve and maintain a safe environment for all people receiving health care.
3. To provide and update information concerning the importance of a safe environment and its effects on daily living.

Assessment

1. Note any dangers and health hazards in the environment of patients, visitors and staff. Recognise the special needs of those who are confused or disorientated and who find difficulty in

carrying out activities of daily living which prevent accidents and ill health.

2. Identify any systematic infections which may lead to psychological problems. Pneumonia and hepatitis, for example, are frequently followed by acute/toxic confusional states.
3. Recognise changes in a person that lead to aggressive behaviour towards themselves or towards others, e.g. the depressed, the aggrieved, the psychotic, the bereaved and the physically ill.
4. Identify any factors which may affect the person's ability to protect himself from dangers in his environment. These are numerous and may include sensory defects, physical disability and state of consciousness.
5. Identify any differences in cultures, custom or religious beliefs which may cause different opinions about safety.
6. Identify any potential dangers in a person's environment which may have caused/be causing physiological dysfunction, e.g. toxic materials in the air, water or soil, which could be a possible cause of birth defects, brain dysfunction and cancers.
7. Identify potential dangers to a person, or the carers, from the violent or suicidal patient.
8. Forecast any potential risks associated with planned treatment/intervention, e.g. surgical operations, diagnostic procedures.

Planning

The plan may involve consideration of one or more of the following:

1. Methods of increasing the person's awareness of their environment, and promoting increased adaptability to it, e.g. protection from hazardous situations, education about safety precautions, overcoming physical or mental disability to maintain safety for themselves and others.
2. Sufficient environmental stimulation for all people in care, irrespective of age, in order to reduce any deterioration of brain cell function, which may lead to reduction in the individual's capability in mastering their environment.
3. Special requirements to safeguard the person with sensory loss or deterioration, e.g. special needs for visual or hearing loss, prevention of the effects of heat, cold, pain or pressure and correct labelling of containers for people suffering from smelling and tasting impairment.
4. Methods of prevention of cross infection to the individual or carers by adequate cleanliness, hygiene, ventilation, disinfection, provision of clothing and an adequate screening process.
5. Special methods to prevent violent behaviour by encouraging

the person to express their aggressive drive in a more socially acceptable way.

6. Planning to ensure that the person or his carers are aware of potentially violent situations, e.g. argumentative or suspicious behaviour, and to provide comprehensive education and training for dealing with violence or aggression.
7. Appropriate programmes of education and support for the individual and carers in all aspects of health and safety, e.g. risks of cross infection, health and safety at work and home, contaminated or infectious materials and potentially hazardous situations.
8. Planning to improve relaxation and reduction of stress, if appropriate, in improving health and safety for individuals and staff.

Implementation

1. Maintain health and safety standards for all individuals at all times.
2. Maintain a quiet environment, without undue, unusual or sudden noises.
3. Promote the importance of safety by setting good examples of safe practices.
4. Be aware that one's own behaviour and non-verbal responses can be the root of a non-therapeutic environment and result in a potentially dangerous confrontation.
5. Ensure safe practices in the storage and administration of drugs, chemicals and dangerous substances, according to Health Unit policy.
6. Safeguard against the danger of fires and encourage the use of fire-retardant materials and furniture as widely as possible and ensure fire-fighting training standards are maintained.
7. Maintain a comprehensive method of ensuring that notifiable diseases are reported to the appropriate authority.
8. Maintain all instruments and equipment in good order by liaison with the appropriate personnel.

Evaluation

In evaluating safety care, there are many things to consider and the following should be in the forefront:

1. The physical condition of the person:
   (a) perceptual defects
   (b) mobility.

2. The mental state of the person:
   (a) level of consciousness
   (b) orientation
   (c) aggression
   (d) suicidal state.
3. Careful observation of alarms such as bells, buzzers and lights.
4. Monitoring of correct implementation of safety procedures, and assurance that they are kept up-to-date, e.g. safe administration of oxygen, fire prevention and management, isolation nursing techniques.
5. Safety measures in the home.
6. Safety from mechanical injury.
7. The person's level of knowledge about maintaining his own personal safety.
8. Monitoring of accident reports.

Reference
Maslow, A.H. (1943) A theory of human motivation, *Psychology Review*, **50**, 370–396.

Bibliography
Blackburn, P. (1988) Freedom to wander, *Nursing Times*, December 7, 54.
  (Safety in an electronic monitoring device which may be used to allow elderly, mentally infirm patients to wander freely).
Bradley, M. (1990) Status passage into nursing: undertaking nursing care, *Journal of Advanced Nursing*, December 1363.
  (Research findings on how nurses cope with attending to specific personal and social needs of patients, and includes dealing with aggression: most useful is this article's bibliography).
Cadwallader, H. (1989) Setting the seal on standards, *Nursing Times (Journal of Infection Control Nursing)*, 13 September, 71.
  (Study in establishing a quality assurance programme for safety for patients and staff in hospital: includes infection control).
HMSO (1988) *Furniture and Furnishings*, Fire Safety Statutory Instrument, London.
Hodgkinson, P. (1980) Psychological approaches to violence, *Nursing Times*, **76**, 1399–1401.
Jackson, M. (1987) The elderly: high risk surgical patients, *Professional Nurse*, **2**, 8, 263–266.
Ricks, E. (1986) A safe and happy refuge, *Geriatric Nursing*, **6**, 2, 32.
Roche, E. (1987) Ethical decisions in nursing, *Professional Nurse*, **2**, 6, 164–166.
Roper, N., Logan, W.W. and Tierney, A.J. (1990) *Elements of Nursing* (3rd Edn), Churchill Livingstone, Edinburgh, pp 83–107.

Rest and sleep

Introduction

Sleep takes up about a third of our lives. Careful studies indicate that it is a time for growth in children and for restoration in all. Psychological effects of sleep deprivation include incoherence, disorientation, and even hallucinations.

Sufficient sleep is essential to health.

Resting includes the art of relaxation, contentment and peace of mind.

Sleeping and resting are taken for granted by people until they are deprived of them by pain, unhappiness, tension or the necessity of staying awake. Enabling an individual to have adequate rest and sleep is a challenge to the nurse.

Aim

To achieve, for each individual, a sleep and rest pattern which is as close to normal as possible and which promotes the optimum state of physical and mental well being for that person.

Assessment

1. Identify the normal sleeping, waking and daytime resting pattern for each individual.
2. Establish what is the normal pre-sleep ritual.
3. Identify those patients with sleeping difficulty and note the cause, e.g. anxiety, mood disturbance, grief, pain, noise, light, cold, heat, hunger and thirst.
4. Establish the individual's preferred posture for sleeping.
5. Assess the need, and resources available, for relatives and others to stay the night.

Planning

The plan may involve consideration of one or more of the following:

1. Planned continuation of a person's normal pattern of rest and sleep where this is compatible with medical and social needs.
2. Inclusion of any important bedtime rituals which are likely to help towards normal sleep, e.g. bedtime stories, comforters, snacks, drinks, reading, music, a night-light.
3. Planned treatments and procedures to occur so that rest and sleep are not unnecessarily disturbed.
4. Designing an adequate and appropriate daytime stimulation programme for people in whom regular daytime sleeping is detrimental to a normal sleeping pattern.
5. Identifying requirements for total pain relief wherever possible so that good rest and sleep are enjoyed fully.

Implementation

1. Be observant for the patient who lies awake and distressed during the night and provide the opportunity for counselling, physical comforts and relief of anxiety during this lonely time.
2. Provide adequate warmth and comfort by the use of suitable bed coverings, appliances and night attire to maximise the possibility of a good sleep pattern.
3. Use pre-sleep relaxation techniques if desired by the wakeful person.
4. Ensure that noise levels and night-lights provide minimum disturbance to the sleep pattern.
5. Give adequate explanation to patients whose sleep must be disturbed by clinical procedures and provide undisturbed rest at another time.
6. Relieve coughing, vomiting, cramp and other physical discomforts which prevent sleep in the individual and other patients.
7. Administer night sedation only when all other avenues of sleep preparation have been explored but found unsuccessful, and observe its after effects. (Such medication should not be withheld at all costs in the mistaken belief that it is always harmful.)

Evaluation

Evaluation of sleeping and resting may involve one or more of the following:

1. Patient's level of satisfaction with the quantity and quality of sleep and rest.
2. Observation of sleep and rest patterns by both day and night staff.

3. The effects, if any, of night sedation.
4. The presence or absence of pain or any other discomforts which may affect sleep.

Bibliography

Boomer, H. and Deakin, A. (1991) Getting children to sleep, *Nursing Times*, 20 March, 40.
(Study into the work of a clinic for children with sleeping difficulties: it contains helpful information about the methods used).

Canavan, T. (1984) The psychobiology of sleep, *Nursing*, **2**, 23, 682–683.

Dorociak, Y. (1990) Aspects of sleep, *Nursing Times*, 19 December, 38–40.
(Information about how sleep affects physical and mental health).

Hayter, J. (1986) Advances in sleep research: implications for nursing practice, *Clinical Nursing Practice*, **14**, 21–45.

Horne, L.A. (1991) No more wakeful nights, *Professional Nurse*, **6**, 7, 383–385.
(Range of practical steps which can be taken to improve sleep for elderly: includes recommendations about complementary therapies which can help with sleep problems).

Morgan, K. (1987) *Sleep and Ageing*, Croom Helm Ltd, Kent.
(Research into both sleep and social gerontology informs this book: offers advice about alternatives to drug induced sleep).

Roper, N., Logan, W.W. and Tierney, A. (1990) *The Elements of Nursing* (3rd Edn), Churchill Livingstone, Edinburgh, pp 315–329.

Religion

Introduction
Man feels a need to relate to the supernatural and to provide explanations for the inexplicable aspects of the universe. To fulfil this need he may turn to religion and the mystic. Supernatural beliefs, with endless variety, are present in every known society. Religion is concerned with thought patterns, beliefs and rituals and is significant in man's attitudes and behaviours.

For centuries it has been part of the ethical code of medical workers to serve the individual without regard to race, creed or colour. Sometimes a person's values in life change with illness. They focus on spiritual beliefs for accepting their illness and planning their future. In this respect, nurses must provide help and guidance that can fulfil this purpose for the person's well being.

Aims
1. To provide such facilities as are required to allow complete freedom of choice to every person to practise their religion.
2. To help people conform to their personal concepts of right and wrong.

Assessment
1. Discuss with the person the need for religious contact in any form.
2. Identify any specific rites and customs related to the individual's daily activities or care following death, e.g., eating, washing, clothing, worshipping, care of the body.
3. Assess facilities required to allow religious beliefs and practices to continue.

In relation to assessment of the individual's religious beliefs, it may be important to discuss the personal and religious beliefs of members of staff, with regard to particular nursing and medical practices.

Planning

The plan may involve consideration of one or more of the following:

1. Provision of facilities and planning for involvement of appropriate personnel for the individual to maintain his religious practices and associated customs.
2. Specific planning to maintain diet, hygiene practices, religious holidays and celebrations.
3. Involvement of family and friends, in the practice of religious customs.
4. Protection of the person from unnecessary harassment because of religious practices.

Implementation

1. Provide opportunities for the person to discuss with others, or receive instruction, if desired, on moral or religious issues.
2. Allow leaders of all religious groups free access to their respective members in promoting religion and customs.
3. Assist the person, family and friends to find comfort and solace through contact with spiritual leaders, if desired in times of crisis, e.g. critical illness, major surgery or bereavement.
4. Accept religious practices and associated rituals in order to prevent unnecessary pain and anguish to the individual.
5. Allow discussion and instruction amongst staff on moral or religious issues which may cause a crisis of conscience in relation to health care practices, e.g. termination of pregnancy, administration of electroconvulsive therapy are two of many matters which may cause controversy.

Evaluation

To evaluate the effectiveness of religious practices and customs the following should be noted:

1. The degree of satisfaction and well-being of the person.
2. The suitability of facilities and environment available for continuing with worship and religious practices.
3. The level of satisfaction of family and friends with the help and support which are provided.

Bibliography

Berkovits, B. (1988) *A Guide to Jewish Practice for Nurses and Medical Staff*, Beth Dinheaflet, 9, London, Court of the Chief Rabbi.

Berkovits, B. (1990) A Jewish perspective on nursing, *Nursing Standard*, 4 April, 32–34.

Burnard, P. (1987) Spiritual distress and the nursing response: theoretical considerations and counselling skills, *Journal of Advanced Nursing*, **12**, 3, 377–382.

Burnard, P. (1990) Learning to care for the spirit, *Nursing Standard*, 24 January, 38–39.
(This article looks at the spiritual domain of the person and considers patients' spiritual needs which, the author believes, are not catered for very well by the nursing profession).

Hay, D. (1987) *Exploring Inner Space* (2nd Edn), Mowbray, London.
(Evidence about the phenomenon of religious experience which the author describes as being more widespread in Britain than is thought likely).

Heywood-Jones, I. (1984) Strictly Kosher, *Nursing Times*, **86**, 4, 61–62.

Heywood-Jones, I. (1984) Ministering angel, *Nursing Times*, **80**, 5, 39.

Heywood-Jones, I. (1984) Bearing witness, *Nursing Times*, **80**, 6, 47–48.

Heywood-Jones, I. (1984) A Punjabi perspective, *Nursing Times*, **80**, 8, 39.

Heywood-Jones, I. (1984) Nursing on the sabbath, *Nursing Times*, **80**, 9, 47.

Males, J. and Boswell, C. (1990) Spiritual needs of people with a mental handicap, *Nursing Standard*, 22 August, 35–37.

Morrison, R. (1990) Spiritual health care and the nurse, *Nursing Standard*, 24 October, 34–35.
(The author is a hospital chaplain, and presents three short care studies to illustrate how nursing to meet spiritual needs can lead to improvement in patients' physical health).

Neuberger, J. (1987) *Caring for Dying People of Different Faiths*, Austen Cornish Publishers Ltd.

Sampson, C. (1982) *The Neglected Ethic: Religious and Cultural Factors in the Care of Patients*, McGraw-Hill, New York.

Occupation

Introduction
For those in paid employment, work provides the financial basis for independence. A person's ability to exercise control and choice in many activities of living is closely related to income.

Whether in paid employment or not, a person's work or productive occupation is a major part of their identity, sense of worth and fulfilment. Society often estimates the individual's value in terms of the work they do.

A person's work, or lack of it, may have profound effects on their physical and mental well-being; conversely, physical and mental well-being significantly affects the work one is able to do. For some, the distinction between work and recreation is subjective, but its relationship to health remains the same.

Aims
1. To help the individual understand the effects of work or productive occupation on physical and mental health.
2. To assist the individual, when appropriate, to engage in work or productive occupation.

Assessment
1. Discuss with the person the effects that health problems may have on their work.
2. Assess the effect of work on the individual, e.g. when a person immerses himself in work exclusively, he may deprive himself of meaningful interpersonal relationships and leisure activities.
3. Assess with the person and relevant members of the multidisciplinary team, the need for work or productive occupation (e.g., people with learning disability who attend Social Education Centres).

4. Identify any particular religious and cultural beliefs of the person. Certain occupations may be offensive and cause distress.

Planning

The plan may involve consideration of one or more of the following:

1. Provision of the necessary stimulus and environment, where possible, to enable active participation in a training or retraining programme following illness.
2. Involvement of all members of the health care team in planning referrals to specialist outside agencies to prepare for the person's future employment.
3. Provision of training advice in matters such as Health and Safety at Work Act, taxes, pension and the law, with regard to future employment.
4. Discussion and planning of possible future employment for people with physical or mental disability by referral to agencies which provide assistance.
5. Provision of privacy for an individual to be interviewed regarding future working arrangements.
6. Pre-retirement preparation, if appropriate.

Implementation

1. Help the person pursue a suitable and meaningful occupation which is appropriate for their capabilities.
2. Encourage the person to use their natural talents where appropriate, either for primary occupation or productive leisure. This is useful in promoting self-satisfaction and self-esteem.
3. Encourage social interactions of people with similar tastes and skills. This may help in preventing loneliness or boredom and the promotion of a 'support system'.
4. Encourage the retention of self-respect, dignity and optimism in the face of unemployment.
5. Offer counselling to those for whom retirement will remove a sense of purpose from their lives.
6. Discourage prejudice and negative attitudes towards people with learning or physical disability in relation to employment and productive occupation.

Evaluation

The following should be taken into consideration:

1. The attitude of the person to the programme of work or occupation activities undertaken.

2. The physical and psychological effects of the activities, and the ability of the person to cope with them.
3. The suitability of the environment and resources used.
4. Discussion with other professionals about the progress towards preparation for work.
5. The level of knowledge and understanding by the person and family about the help which is available.

Bibliography

Hall, E.M. (1979) Helping the patient with work or productive occupation, *Nursing Times*, 21st June, 1061–1062.

Littler, C.R. (1985) *The Experience of Work*, Gower, London.

Royal College of Nursing (1983) The nurse's contribution to the health of the worker, *Report of the Nursing Commission*, Permanent Commission and International Association on Occupational Health. R.C.N., London

Roper, N., Logan, W. and Tierney, A. (1990) *The Elements of Nursing* (3rd Edn) Churchill Livingstone, Edinburgh, pp 274–292.

Smith, R. (1987) *Unemployment and Health: a Disaster and a Challenge*, Oxford University Press, Oxford.

Willson, M. (1987) *Occupational Therapy in Long-Term Psychiatry* (2nd Edn) Churchill Livingstone, Edinburgh, pp 164–190.

(Theory and practice of preparing patients for productive occupation on discharge from care, or whilst receiving long-term care: written predominantly for occupational therapists, but useful reading for all health care workers).

Recreation and play

Introduction

Recreation and play refer to fun or doing things to pass the time pleasantly. The nature, and perhaps the purpose, of play changes as a person becomes older. Recreation forms an important part of a person's social, psychological and physical growth. Developmental sequences of recreation and play activities can be identified.

Everyone plays. Play continues as a normal activity from childhood to old age. Enjoyment is a prime objective in all forms of play, whether it is performed for relaxation, competition, entertainment or development. Recreation is used as a form of therapy in three ways: to study a person's behaviour; as a means of expressing inner feelings; and, with frequent practice, to develop skills.

Aims

Recreation and play in health care settings aim to:

1. Give enjoyment, fulfilment and generally enhance the quality of life.
2. Promote physical, psychological, social and cognitive development.
3. Provide therapy.
4. Promote relaxation.

Assessment

1. Ascertain the need for physical, psychological and social development through recreation and play.
2. Consider the availability of facilities for recreation and play both in the hospital and in the community.
3. Identify the difficulties a disabled person faces in gaining access to premises for recreational activities.

4. Identify the specific difficulties a person has in being able to play, e.g. physical and sensory handicaps, finance and facilities, companionship, time and motivation.
5. Assess the influence of culture, age and sex on the acceptability of planned activities to individuals (e.g. not everyone likes Bingo).
6. Assess the levels and types of play of which the individual is capable.
7. Identify the preferences of the individual for play and recreation.

Planning

The plan may involve consideration of one or more of the following:

1. Negotiation, with the person, of appropriate periods during his day for play and recreation.
2. Provision of adequate space, toys and equipment.
3. Consideration of safety, both in the choice and use of equipment and environment, and of the acceptable level of risk in undertaking activities.
4. Planning for rehabilitation exercises, requiring effort and repetition, to learn new skills.
5. Involvement, where appropriate, of other members of the multidisciplinary team (e.g. physiotherapist, occupational therapist, play therapist, speech therapist, psychologist), in planning therapeutic play.

Implementation

1. Observe those participating in play or recreation for signs of fatigue, boredom, frustration or overexcitement and recognise when to intervene with advice.
2. Be aware of the effects of recreational and play activities on those nearby who are not participating.
3. Ensure that other basic needs are not neglected during the pursuit of play/recreation and that play/recreation is not unnecessarily disrupted by routine care.
4. Check and maintain the state of repair and hygiene of toys and equipment to prevent injury and cross infection.
5. Organise compatible groups for play and recreation, which an individual may attend if desired.
6. Involve relatives and friends as appropriate.

Evaluation

The following points may be considered:

1. The person's level of satisfaction with recreation/play provided.
2. The effects of play on the person's physical and mental condition.
3. Checking if therapeutic goals are being achieved.
4. The suitability of the physical environment and other resources for play and recreation.
5. The motivation and capability of the person to engage in play activities.
6. The level of understanding of the individual about the benefits of recreation to physical and mental well-being.

Bibliography

Carlisle, D. (1991) The state of the art, *Nursing Times*, 19th June, 50–51.
(Survey of arts activities in the Health Service, with contact names for further information).

Croucher, N. (1981) *Outdoor Pursuits for Disabled People*, Woodhead-Faulkner Ltd., Cambridge.

Elliott, V. and Milne, D. (1991) Patient's best friend? *Nursing Times*, 6th February, 34–35.
(Report which assesses the benefits of introducing pets into a care of the elderly ward).

McBey, M.A. (1985) The therapeutic aspects of gardens and gardening; an aspect of total patient care. *Journal of Advanced Nursing*, **10**, 6, 591–595.

Roper, N., Logan, W. and Tierney, A. (1990) *Elements of Nursing* (3rd Edn), Churchill Livingstone, Edinburgh.

Sutherland, A. and Soames, P. (1984) *Adventure Play with Handicapped Children*, Souvenir Press, London.

Thompson, J. (1990) Playing at work, *Community Outlook*, April, 15–18.
(Importance of play in child development).

Weller, B.F. (1980) *Helping Sick Children Play*, Baillière Tindall, London.

Willson, M. (1987) *Occupational Therapy in Long-Term Psychiatry* (2nd Edn), Churchill Livingstone, Edinburgh.

Learning

Introduction

Learning has been described as 'a change in behaviour, more or less persistent in nature, which is brought about by activity, observation or experience'.

Learning is a lifelong process beginning in infancy by means of play and continuing by formal and informal experience, into old age. Through learning one acquires or modifies knowledge, attitudes, psychomotor skills, social and interpersonal skills, emotions, roles, habits and self-concept.

By learning one may become more understanding of and well adjusted to one's environment and circumstances, and thereby be more independent and able to live a fulfilling life; on the other hand, one may learn faulty behaviour leading to ill health of a physical, mental or social nature, becoming more dependent, poorly adjusted, and even hurtful to others.

Some people become dependent on caring professionals as a result of a lack of learning or by learning bad habits (e.g. poor hygiene, inadequate safety measures). Such conditions must be cured, ameliorated or at least prevented from becoming worse by helping patients learn correctly.

Preventative medicine depends largely on health education and the ability, opportunity and willingness of individuals to learn how to control their own health and that of others by adjusting their behaviour or environment.

Disability of any nature, whether permanent or temporary, is less likely to reduce the quality of the lives of individuals when they can learn to overcome the obstacles their handicap presents. Habilitation and rehabilitation are key concepts in all fields of nursing.

Sometimes learning is the main component of the person's treatment and takes the form of highly specialised techniques such as psychotherapy, behaviour modification, group therapy, therapeutic community, social and interpersonal skills training. These are particularly relevant (though not exclusively so) for people with mental illness and learning disability, where maladaptive learning or learning difficulties may be major factors in the patient's condition.

Aims

1. To enable a person to achieve that degree of learning necessary for maximum independence and maximum fulfilment.
2. To help families and friends of the person to support the learning process.

Assessment

1. Identify the ways in which the individual perceives himself and his ability to learn.
2. Determine the person's willingness to learn and be aware of those factors which will promote motivation for learning.
3. Agree with the person, family and all members of the caring team, where appropriate, on what needs to be learnt and priorities for learning.
4. Find out whether or not a person has any specific handicap or learning disability, e.g. poor memory, sensory handicap, other physical, psychological or cognitive difficulty.
5. Assess the person's expectations with regard to learning ability and outcome of learning.
6. Elicit the person's present level of knowledge and skill in preparation for a specific learning programme.
7. Seek information regarding the situation in which new learning will be used (e.g. the person's home, social environment, pattern of life).
8. Analyse whether or not new learning is appropriate for the person and whether the environment or the behaviour of nurses and others may be factors which need alteration.

Planning

The plan may involve consideration of one or more of the following:

1. The time and resources available for helping the person to learn, before setting what is a realistic goal.
2. Clarification, with the person and/or his family, of the reasons behind any learning or retraining programme which is to be planned.

3. Negotiation of realistic and achievable goals for learning, with the person and/or his family.
4. Making a contract with the person and/or his family, about a target date for achieving learning objectives.
5. Liaison with other health care professionals during the preparation of learning and retraining programmes, to ensure that all teaching is co-ordinated and compatible with any other treatment being received.
6. Careful consideration of whether or not any learning programme will significantly improve the quality of life of an individual, particularly when that individual is unable to communicate their wants and needs. Occasionally this may need referral to an independent advocate.

Implementation

1. Ensure that the place of learning is free from distractions.
2. Be aware that anxiety, pain and tiredness are barriers to effective learning and reduce the effects of these in order to pursue programmes for learning or training, or postpone a training session until a more appropriate time.
3. Use effectively those resources available to help patients learn, e.g. specialist organisations, health education literature, toys, television, libraries, other professionals.
4. Maintain accurate records of progress in learning, so that the person is not subject to gaps in learning, or to unnecessary repetition.
5. Allow flexibility in the implementation of learning programmes so that any necessary changes may be made when discovered by regular evaluation.
6. Utilise the person's positive motivating factors identified during assessments, to reinforce his efforts.
7. Ensure that the person has the opportunity to practise new skills, or to recall information, until both he and the nurse are satisfied that the intended goal has been achieved.

Evaluation

The following points may be considered:

1. Observe whether or not a significant and beneficial change in the person's behaviour or state of mind has occurred, in accordance with stated goals.
2. Elicit from the person or his family a critical appraisal of the method used to help him learn, and the value of what has been learned.

3. Record for future reference the success or failure of approaches used to help the person learn.
4. Ask the person and/or family how helpful and accessible they found the resources recommended to them and assist them to make further enquiries if necessary.
5. Discuss with colleagues and other members of the caring team those factors which helped or hindered the learning process and use this information in future programme design.

Bibliography

Brandon, D. (1990) Gentle teaching, *Nursing Times*, 10th January, 62–63.
('Gentle teaching', a successful method of helping people with learning disability to learn and progress is described. The main issue in the article is to challenge staff to work as partners with the clients rather than to dominate them).

Cohen, S.A. (1981) Patient education: a review of the literature, *Journal of Advanced Nursing*, 6, 1, 11–18.

Coutts, L. and Hardy, L. (1985) *Teaching for Health: The Nurse as Health Educator*, Churchill Livingstone, Edinburgh.

Fletcher, V. (1987) An individualised teaching programme, following primary uncomplicated myocardial infarction, *Journal of Advanced Nursing*, 12, 2, 195–200.

McGee, J. (1990) Gentle teaching: the basic tenet, *Nursing Times*, 8th August, 68–72.
(Report on a study in applying 'gentle teaching' to a group of 15 people who displayed aggressive and life-threatening behaviour).

Redman, B.K. (1984) *The Process of Patient Teaching in Nursing* (5th Edn), C.V. Mosby Co., St. Louis, USA.

Sugden, J. (1985) The psychiatric treatment setting: some general considerations, *Psychiatric Nursing: Recent Advances in Nursing*, 12, Churchill Livingstone, Edinburgh, pp 1–17.
(On therapeutic environment for living and learning).

Tilley, J.D., Gregor, F.M. and Thiessen, V. (1987) The nurse's role in patient education: incongruent perceptions among nurses and patients, *Journal of Advanced Nursing*, 12, 3, 291–302.

Turnbull, J. (1990) The emperor's new clothes? *Nursing Times*, 8th August, 64–66.
(Critical appraisal of 'gentle teaching' for people with learning disability and disruptive behaviour problems).

Valletuti, P.J. (1983) *Severely and Profoundly Handicapped Students: Their Nature and Needs*, P.H. Brooks, USA.

Wilson-Barnett, J. (1983) *Patient Teaching: Recent Advances in Nursing*, 6, Churchill Livingstone, Edinburgh.

Wilson-Barnett, J. and Osborne, J. (1983) Studies evaluating patient teaching: implications for practice, *International Journal of Nursing Studies*, 20, 1, 33–44.

Expressing sexuality

Introduction

Expression of sexuality begins at birth when, in most cultures, the selection of names, clothing and the association of certain colours is performed by parents. Throughout life, dressing and grooming remain important in expressing sexuality.

Most children gradually become aware of gender and may imitate sex-typed roles defined by family and society. As they mature they may choose to identify with, or reject, such roles or stereotypes and exercise personal preferences in their expression of sexuality.

At puberty everyone has to come to terms with physical and emotional changes which, for many, can be stressful.

In adolescence and adulthood the patterns of one's sexual relationships, attitudes, values and preferences develop and these are personal to the individual and should be respected.

At any time in life, physical, psychological and social problems may have a profound effect on a person's expression of sexuality. This should be taken into account when it involves a person's health or the delivery of care.

People who do not have an active sex life still express sexuality in their clothes, grooming, activities and roles.

Aims

1. To help the person to achieve an acceptable level of sexual expression, according to the special circumstances relating to health care provision.
2. To provide guidance, information and support to the person, and significant others, if sexual or personal difficulties exist.

Assessment

This may include any of the following:

1. Appreciate the embarrassment and anxiety to both the receiver and the giver of care during intimate procedures.
2. When appropriate, assess the person's stage of sexual development.
3. Ascertain the individual's needs to express sexuality by appearance, general behaviour and communication.
4. Ascertain any specific problems that an individual may have in expressing sexuality and which he wishes to overcome.
5. Identify the potential effects of medical and surgical intervention and their influences on the individual's ability to express sexuality, e.g. disfiguring surgery, cardiopulmonary disorders, drugs.
6. Assess the sociological, cultural and religious influences on attitudes towards the expression of sexuality.
7. Identify any anxieties caused by long-term separations from spouse or partner.
8. Check the possibility of limitations of the person's environment on expressing sexuality.
9. Observe for signs of sexual expression which may be socially unacceptable, generally, and therefore a potential barrier to healthy interpersonal relationships, e.g. public masturbation, or inappropriate behaviour for a person's age, which may occur as a consequence of learning disability or mental disorder.

Planning

The plan may involve consideration of one or more of the following:

1. Respect the embarrassment and anxiety to both the receiver and the giver of care during intimate procedures.
2. The pattern of the day, and provision of the best environment, to minimise the effects of illness or hospitalisation on the person's normal sexual relationships, e.g. privacy, double beds, comfort.
3. Programme of education about sexual development, sexual activity, preventing sexually-transmitted diseases, where appropriate, e.g. the person with learning disability may need supportive education.
4. Planned therapy and support for the person with particular sexual difficulty, in association with psychotherapists, and/or specialists in helping the physically disabled in sexual expression.

5. Planned use of additional facilities to enhance sexual expression, e.g. hairdressing, grooming, health and fitness programmes.

Implementation

1. Communicate skilfully to preserve the person's self-esteem.
2. Safeguard confidentiality and privacy in matters pertaining to a person's sexuality.
3. Be sensitive to signs of anxiety and embarrassment when dealing with aspects of sexuality.
4. Help the person come to terms with possible changes regarding the expression of sexuality as a result of illness or the effects of drugs.
5. Promote acceptance of sexual expression as part of daily living to Health Care Workers and others who may give significant support to the person receiving help.

Evaluation

One or more of the following may be involved in evaluating the ability to express sexuality.

1. Discussion with the person about feelings and attitudes towards sexual expression.
2. The effectiveness of care given to relieve any pain, anxiety or discomforts which may have been associated with sexual activity.
3. The person's knowledge and understanding about coping with sexuality and maintaining complete health in this activity.
4. Discussion with other therapists about the outcomes of care.
5. The suitability of the environment for continuing sexual activity.

Bibliography

Allen, I. (1987) *Education in Sex and Personal Relationships*, P.S.I. Research Report No. 665, Pinter Publishers Ltd, Oxford.
(Major study about the attitudes of various groups in society towards sex education).

Carolan, C. (1984) Handicap – less important than loving, *Nursing Times*, **80**, 39, 28–30.

Cochrane, M. (1984) Immaculate infection, *Nursing Times*, **80**, 39, 31–32.
(For information on sexual problems faced by those with rheumatoid arthritis).

Dawson-Shepperd, R. (1984) When the carpet is no longer big enough, *Nursing Times*, **80**, 39, 33–34.
(For information on sexual needs of the disabled).

Greengross, W. (1976) *Entitled to Love*, Malaby Press Ltd, London.
(The sexual and emotional needs of the handicapped).

Roper, N., Logan, W. and Tierney, A. (1990) *The Elements of Nursing* (3rd Edn), Churchill Livingstone, Edinburgh, pp 304–314.

Savage, J. (1987) *Nurses, Gender and Sexuality,* Heinemann Medical Books, London, pp 141–156.

(Provides clear guidance in the sort of sexual health care which nurses should aim to provide: the rest of the book addresses nurses and their own sexuality).

Savage, J. (1990) Sexuality and nursing care: setting the scene, *Nursing Standard,* 6th June, 24–25.

(First of a major series of articles in *Nursing Standard* during 1990).

Skrine, R.L. (Ed.) (1989) *Introduction to Psychosexual Medicine,* Montana Press, Carlisle.

(Ten authors with long experience of working with psychosexual difficulties describe their work, and the theory and practice of their treatments).

Webb, C. (1985) *Sexuality, Nursing and Health,* J. Wiley and Sons Ltd, Sussex.

Pain

Introduction

A contemporary clinical definition of pain is 'a more or less localised sensation of discomfort, distress or agony, resulting from the stimulation of specialised nerve endings'. Pain has an important function as a body defence mechanism: it induces the individual to move away from the source and it may be a useful diagnostic feature. But it can become unhelpful and destructive.

Pain is a highly subjective phenomenon. Admission, acceptance and expression of pain are influenced by a person's social attitudes and culture. It is not enough to say that pain is a result of disease, injury or malfunction, and that the degree of pain felt is proportional to the extent of injury or disease. Quite severe pain can be felt by people who have no organic reason for pain: this pain is not imaginary but is felt very strongly. Similarly any relationship between the pain felt and the level of injury is refuted by the phenomenon of mystics who walk through hot embers without experiencing pain, or disturbed persons who indulge in self-mutilation for relief of tension but who feel no pain.

Pain is often classified as acute (or transient) or chronic (persistent) pain. Acute pain, e.g. that experienced in renal colic or myocardial infarction, is a warning that something harmful is happening. It is usually well localised although it may be severe and frightening. An accurate description of the pain is an essential and helpful diagnostic tool. Being able to discuss the cause of the expected transient nature of the pain can, itself, aid relief for the person. In contrast, chronic pain, not a passing event, is a much more threatening experience. This sort of pain is usually much less localised, burning, throbbing, or aching in character, and since no physical reaction is effective in removing the painful stimulus, the pain tends to get worse rather than better. Both types of pain may coexist in the same individual.

Pain has physiological, psychological and sociological dimensions, but, no matter what the underlying cause, pain is what the person feels.

Aim

To strive, intelligently and compassionately, with all other members of the caring team, to achieve complete relief of pain in order to improve quality of life in any circumstance, for any individual who is experiencing pain.

Assessment

1. Specify accurately, through discussion with and observation of the patient, the location, onset, severity and nature of the pain. (In some cases individual rating scales may be useful in assessing and reassessing a person's pain.)
2. Acknowledge that pain without apparent organic cause is, nevertheless, real to the person and worthy of serious consideration.
3. Identify the presence and cause of any anxiety and distress in the person with pain.
4. Be considerate of those individuals, especially young children, people with learning disability and the disorientated, who are unable to communicate their pain verbally, and observe for the expression of pain by other means, e.g. crying, changed behaviour, facial expression, immobility, guarding of a painful area.
5. Assessment of any change of personality which is caused by chronic pain.
6. Identification of those factors, including cultural ones, which affect an individual's expression of pain, or his ability to cope with it.
7. Assessment of any precipitating factors which stimulate the sensation of pain, e.g. real, threatened or fantasised loss, guilt, aggression, forbidden feelings, depression, loss of self-esteem.
8. Identification of the special needs of some individuals who enjoy pain, sometimes self-inflicted, because of the psychological reward it may bring, e.g. receipt of attention, relief of guilt, sexual excitement.

Planning

The plan may involve consideration of one or more of the following:

1. Ensuring that the individual is made aware of a potentially painful experience induced by operations, procedures, etc., in order to allow a measure of self-control over the pain experience, and to reduce feelings of anxiety and failure if pain is experienced.
2. Planning, with the person whenever possible, the possible pain-relieving methods to be used, their duration and effects, so

that the person knows there is an end to pain in sight. (Other professionals in the care team may be involved in this aspect of planning.)

3. The use of methods to minimise all other physical discomforts which may exacerbate pain, e.g. bad positioning, constipation, vomiting, dyspnoea, inappropriate clothing, poor hygiene, skin and mucous membrane irritation, badly applied wound dressings, abnormal body temperature.

4. Provision of a sympathetic therapeutic climate in which individuals can learn about their pain, and the vocabulary which may be used to express it.

5. Planning to allow the individual to control the timing and process of potentially painful procedures, if they so wish, in order to reduce the fear and stress of such events (especially important for children).

6. Provision of psychological support and information to the family and friends of the individual in pain, so that they understand that pain may cause profound changes of personality. By learning to accept this they can continue to provide vital support and contact for the individual.

7. Teaching and giving accurate information to the person, family and friends, about pain-relieving drugs which are recommended, e.g. sedation and loss of interest are not necessary accompaniments to adequate pain control.

Implementation

1. Introduce appropriate pain-relieving measures with the person's informed consent.

   Examples – therapeutic touch, massage, skin vibration
   - variation in positioning
   - splintering of limbs
   - traction
   - hot and cold local applications
   - low voltage transcutaneous stimulation
   - hypnosis
   - acupunture
   - relaxation
   - distraction
   - inhalations (e.g. Entonox)
   - radiotherapy
   - neurosurgery and nerve blocks
   - diet
   - spiritual support

2. Use relevant strategies to ensure that pain-seeking behaviours do not become the last resort of the person.

3. Provide skilled counselling, particularly for people with intractable pain, where empathy and time for listening may provide some relief for feelings of anger, frustration and despair.
4. Be meticulous in the administration of pain-relieving medication, according to the individual's drug regime, and observe and report its effectiveness and any undesirable side effects.
5. Appreciate that pain in the child provokes crying which elicits comfort from the parent. Relief of pain resulting in pleasure may be equated by reunion with a loved object.
6. Support the person who is going through a painful psychological experience associated with daily living.

Evaluation

Evaluation should be a continuous process and its timing will depend on the needs of the individual. Wherever possible involve that individual, because he is the only person able to judge the success or failure of pain control.

The following should be considered:

1. Use of pain evaluation charts, e.g. pain thermometer.
2. Listening to and observing the person and his response to all pain control measures in use.
3. Effects and side effects of drugs on the physical and mental state of the person.
4. Discussion with family, friends and other carers.
5. The knowledge and understanding of the patient and family about the pain, and its relief.
6. The general physical and mental state of the person.

Bibliography

Broom, A. and Jellicoe, H. (1987) *Living with your Pain: A Guide to Managing Pain*, BPS/Methuen, Leicester.
Copp, L.A. (1985) Perspectives on pain, *Recent Advances in Nursing*, **11**, Churchill Livingstone, Edinburgh.
Copp, L.A. (1990) The spectrum of suffering, *American Journal of Nursing*, August, 35–39.
(Described in the journal as a timeless classic which was first published in 1974: 148 people were interviewed to find out how they described their pain and coped with it. Implications for patient care are listed clearly at the end of the article).
Gartside, G. (1986) Alternative methods of pain relief, *Nursing: The Add-on Journal of Clinical Nursing*, **3**, 11, 405–407.
Gaston-Johansson, F. and Asklund-Gustaisson, M. (1985) A baseline study for the development of an instrument for the assessment of pain, *Journal of Advanced Nursing*, **10**, 6, 539–546.
Hayward, J. (1973) *Information: A Prescription Against Pain*, R.C.N. London.

Hosking, J. and Weichew, E. (1985) Post-Operative Pain – Understanding its Nature and How to Treat it, Faber and Faber, London, pp 14–15.
(Assessment of pain); pp.146–149 (achieving analgesia without drugs).

Hough, A. (1986) Handling the patient in pain, *Nursing Times*, **82**, 15, 28–31.

Hunter, D. (1991) Relief through teamwork, *Nursing Times*, 24 April, 35–38.
(Report about the effects of setting up an Acute Pain Service team in one hospital: formal assessment of pain is important, advanced methods of pain relief are now in use in general and surgical wards, with traditional methods being questioned by both medical and nursing staff).

Jerrett, M. and Evans, K. (1986) Children's pain vocabulary, *Journal of Advanced Nursing*, **11**, 4, 403–408.

Latham, J. (1991) *Pain Control* (2nd Edn), Austen Cornish, London.
(Excellent small book, designed for practical use by everyone concerned with improving the effectiveness of pain relief).

Melzack, R. and Wall, P.D. (1988) *The Challenge of Pain* (2nd Edn), Penguin, Harmondsworth.

Raiman, J. (1986) Pain relief – a two-way process, *Nursing Times*, **82**, 15, 14–18.

Rodin, J. (1983) *Will this Hurt? Preparing Children for Hospital and Medical Procedures*, R.C.N., London.

Walding, M.F. (1991) Pain, anxiety and powerlessness, *Journal of Advanced Nursing*, **16**, 388–397.
(Review of some substantial literature about factors which affect the pain experience: the author suggests that intensity of pain is reduced when there is a reduced feeling of powerlessness).

Dying and bereavement

'There is general understanding that terminal care refers to the management of the person in whom the advent of death is felt to be certain and
not too far off, and from whom medical effort has turned away from
curative therapy and is concentrated on caring'

J.M. Holford, *Care of the Dying*
1973 National Symposium, DHSS London

During this time, the nurse should be able to provide skilled support
to meet the emotional, spiritual and physical needs of the dying
person, the family, and other members of their social group. The
smallest things may assume great significance, and meticulous
attention to minute detail is essential. There should also be recog-
nition of, and support to meet, the needs of colleagues who are
involved in caring for dying people.

Not all death is expected or timely. The families and loved ones of
those who have died suddenly (e.g. stillborn and cot-death babies,
suicides, trauma victims, myocardial infarction) require special consideration.

Nurses must develop the resources to comfort the bereaved, bear
the sorrow of grieving and help people to face death with dignity.
Above all, the aim should be to develop mutual understanding
between the patient, their relatives and professionals so that fear and
anxiety disappear.

Aim

1. To assist all people in whom death is expected, to achieve a
   peaceful acceptance of death, wherever possible.
2. To provide skilled support and comfort to bereaved relatives,
   friends and fellow patients, whether death has been expected or
   sudden or untimely.
3. To provide support for nurses and other caring professionals

who need specific help to cope with their own feelings associated with death and dying.

Assessment

1. Assess effectively the specific physical symptoms which may be experienced by a dying person, e.g.

    Pain—see Chapter in this book

    Problems with bladder and bowels

    Problems of nutrition and fluid intake

    Problems involving the skin and mucous membranes

    Mouth care

    Respiratory problems

    Problems associated with mobility

    Problems associated with rest and sleep

    Problems of personal hygiene, body odour

    Possible causes need careful identification by detailed assessment, and the person's normal routine should be discussed.

2. Ascertain, through skilled listening, questioning and observation, the degree to which the dying person and family are aware of the diagnosis, and assess their wishes in this respect.

3. Assess the importance of religious practice, worship and ritual which may affect the programme of care for a dying person.

4. Understand the emotional stages experienced by dying people, and demonstrate a sympathetic and confident approach in allowing them to express their feelings of anxiety, denial, bargaining, depression and acceptance.

5. Recognise that sharing of information is essential if all team members are to work well together and derive a sense of satisfaction which can compensate for the emotional stresses of caring for the dying.

6. Provide opportunity and privacy for nurses and other team members to talk over matters of mutual concern, to express emotions and gain support from each other in time of particular difficulty (especially when a death has occurred).

7. Recognise the signs of strain in colleagues, as characterised by fatigue, reluctance to face the day, depression, headaches, dependency on alcohol or other drugs, isolation from the group.

8. Assess the potential for distressing circumstances in which the relatives of potential organ donors may be approached for consent to remove organs at, or soon after, the death of their loved one.

Planning

Specific planning for the care of a dying person may require reference to one or more of the other sections in this book. Additional aspects of planning may include:

1. Provision of a suitable physical environment for the dying person, in accordance with their wishes, which allows them to pursue interests, maintain family and social contacts and which does not restrict desired physical activity.
2. Planning for relatives to be given facilities to attend to their own needs, e.g. meals, sleep, hygiene, privacy and communication.
3. Means of providing physical support to relatives caring for dying people at home, e.g. enlisting help of the Marie Curie Foundation, Social Services, Community Health Care Team.
4. Giving information to families about finance and special equipment to aid nursing at home.
5. Planning for administration and teaching about any medications used (see chapter on pain).
6. Provision of facilities and activities for specific rites and rituals associated with dying and death, for the individual and family.
7. Special consideration of parents of still-born babies, to allow them time and privacy to express their grief and to support each other.
8. The possibility of setting up a patient and relative support group, and the need for referrals, if this is an appropriate move, to provide individuals with a forum to express their feelings and receive mutual support.
9. The possibility of referrals to other professionals, e.g. counsellors, clergy, psychotherapists.
10. The level to which family and friends will be involved in any aspect of care for the dying person, and which is in compliance with that person's wishes.

Implementation

1. Endeavour to act in the best interests of the dying person at all times when treatment methods, or their withdrawal, are the subject of ethical discussion. (The nurse should not opt out of such decision making.)
2. Recognise the right of staff to dissociate themselves from participation in treatment which they consider unethical (e.g. termination of pregnancy).
3. Be prepared to discuss openly and honestly with other patients their questions and fears about the death of their colleague/ friend, without breach of confidentiality.

4. Strive to avoid the barrier of secrecy between nurse and patient, where information about expected death has been withheld, by promoting good multidisciplinary team communication where the contribution of each member, however junior, is valued. In this way, the decision to 'tell', based on a full knowledge of the person involved, may be more easily reached.

5. Enter into full and skilled communication with the person and their family, when they have received information about the expected death, and whenever they request help.

6. Provide relatives with information and contacts for bereavement counselling following the death of their loved one.

7. Assist in the administration of documents and property to the family, after death of the relative, in order to prevent aggravation of inevitable feelings of anxiety, disorganisation and frustration.

8. Prepare the body of a deceased person with dignity and according to any ritual or religious observances of that person.

Evaluation

Traditional approaches to nursing and medical education possibly give prominence to the curative role of the nurse and doctor. Consequently the death of a person may be perceived as professional failure. Evaluation should be concerned with measuring the quality of care delivered until the moment of death, the appropriate management and care of the body, and subsequent care of the bereaved. Therefore preceding evaluations in other sections apply to the care of the dying.

Additional aspects of evaluation might include:

1. Was there intervention, in good time, when signs of strain were apparent, by providing opportunity and personal contact for discussion of difficulties associated with caring for the dying and bereaved?

2. Was an opportunity provided for bereaved relatives to discuss the care that the deceased received and to represent their views to members of the care team?

3. Did members of the caring team discuss to what extent the expressed wishes of the dying person and their relatives were respected? Where such wishes were not complied with, determine if policies and practices require review.

4. Were the views expressed by those people who were in the vicinity of the dying person considered and what action could have been taken to diminish their distress?

5. Was a suitable balance between professional life and personal life achieved by the care team members to relieve continuous

strain and allow them to return refreshed to a stressful situation? (This may require particular attention to off-duty arrangements.)

Bibliography

Conboy-Hill, S. (1986) Their death in your hands, *Professional Nurse*, **2**, 2, 51–53.
(For review of psychological and nursing literature in terminal care).

Cowley, S. (1990) Who qualifies for terminal care? *Nursing Times*, 30 May, 29–31.
(Highlights the plight of people who seem to be deprived of adequate terminal care because they are not dying of cancer: useful reminder that not all terminal care is because of malignant disease).

Field, D. (1984) 'We didn't want him to die on his own'—nurses' accounts of nursing dying patients, *Journal of Advanced Nursing*, **9**, 1, 59–70.
(Particular reference to emotional involvement with dying patients).

Harris, L. (1990) The disadvantaged dying, *Nursing Times*, 30 May, 26–28.

Kennedy, L. (1990) *Euthanasia: the Good Death*, Chatto

Kubler-Ross, E. (1969) *On Death and Dying*, Macmillan, New York.

Lindars, J. (1991) Holistic care in parasuicide, *Nursing Times*, 10 April, 30–31.

Lombardi, T. (1987) Helping clients to come to terms with loss, *Professional Nurse*, **2**, 6, 178–180.

Lunt, B. and Jenkins, J. (1983) Goal-setting in terminal care: a method of recording treatment aims and priorities, *Journal of Advanced Nursing*, **8**, 6, 495–505.

Murray Parkes, C. (1972) *Bereavement Studies of Grief in Adult Life*, Penguin, London.

National Childbirth Trust (1984) *Mothers Writing about the Death of a Baby*, N.C.T., London

Neuberger, J. (1987) *Caring for Dying People of Different Faiths*, Austen Cornish Ltd, London.

Pike, C. (1983) The broken heart syndrome and the elderly patient, *Nursing Times*, **79**, 19, 50–53.

Robbins, J. (Ed.) (1989) *Caring for the Dying Patient and the Family*, Harper and Row, London.
(Covers many different aspects of care including symptom control, nursing people with AIDS, cultural and religious factors, the death of children, home care for dying people).

Ross, T. (1982) Death wish, *Nursing Mirror*, **155**, 18, 19–21.
(About helping the attempted suicide patient).

Saunders, B. (1982) Staff support, *Nursing: The Add-on Journal of Clinical Nursing*, February, 1498–1499.

Speck, P. (1978) *Loss and Grief in Medicine*, Ballière Tindall, Eastbourne.

Trent Regional Health Authority (1988) *No Second Chance: a Discussion Document on the Development of Terminal Care Services*, Trent R.H.A., Sheffield.

Wilkes, E. (Ed.) (1978) *Terminal Care*, Update-Siebert Publications Ltd., Guildford, Surrey.

The concept of integrated care planning

This book is unique in that it describes a process for the delivery of care to patients in those areas which are representative of common basic human needs during illness or disability. This final chapter seeks to demonstrate how to develop multidisciplinary objectives in a single record of care to formalise the participation in care planning by the patient and to propose a model for true multidisciplinary audit.

The nursing profession has endeavoured to perfect care planning and to place the patient, or his relatives, in a position of control demanding a specific regimen of care and treatment in or out of hospital. Nurses have sought to develop 'the care plan' individually, believing that no patient is the same, and that his needs cannot be distilled into a package of procedures available on some shelf ready to be applied with a successful outcome. Thus the nursing process has evolved to include a method of documenting care in all of its planning stages.

This process for documenting care follows a normal pattern of problem solving. It identifies the 'problem' or 'need', states the objective for solving the problem, describes the nursing interventions to achieve that objective, and finally provides an opportunity to evaluate the success of such intervention.

Depending upon the results of the evaluation, the objective may be declared as achieved or it may be amended, and a new set of interventions described. It is therefore a dynamic process, designed to assist a change in direction at any point in the care programme. The quality of care and the standards set are thus measurable if the process is used correctly. If the patient suffers from post-operative complications, for instance, and a schedule of care is designed appropriately, it should lead to relief of problems or enable the unresolved problem to be further addressed by the nurse, or to be taken up by another professional, e.g. a medical officer.

The nursing process as currently used throughout the United Kingdom has been highlighted in the *Clinical Grading Structure* (Department of Health, 1988). Each of the grades from C through to I refers to care planning in some or all of its stages. To qualify at 'Grade C', for instance, the participant must prove that he or she did 'participate' in the "assessing of care needs and implementation of programmes of care." Grade D demands a greater responsibility and states that the nurse must demonstrate that she is "responsible for the assessment of care needs and the development of programmes of care, and/or the implementation and evaluation of these programmes." Similarly, references to care planning become criteria in the more senior grades at an ever increasing level of demand. It could be argued that no other profession has been thus treated and that nurses have been honoured in their long desire for effective delivery of planned care.

This chapter examines the part played by the patient in care planning and explains the need to move from uni-professional planning to a shared approach with relevant disciplines involved in the episode of care.

The patient's role

The patient is not a peripheral player in the daily activities of nurses, but is at the centre of events and the reason why nurses are needed. The questions which need to be asked include – "Is the patient to play a passive role, simply to receive care by those 'who know best'?" or "Is he to be active in the process of planning, gaining access to his notes, owning the agreed plan and actually entering his own objectives into the notes which form the legal prime document, i.e. the total care documentation?" If the latter is agreed then the patient becomes a fully fledged member of the multi-disciplinary team, adopting a suitable position of control over his life events. Of course, it may be that the seriousness of the patient's condition renders him impotent in his contribution, perhaps for the total episode. Wherever possible, though, the patient should be actively involved, but protected from undue stress and responsibility. The nearest relative or the named advocate may equally represent the interests of the patient at certain times.

It would be useful at this point to study the 'audit square' referred to in the Introduction and to consider how this may be adapted in the light of these considerations.

The 'audit square' indicates that the responsibility for care planning lies with the professionals in the multidisciplinary teams and leads to an audit of care-effectiveness with the patient in the passive centre. Perhaps the patient has been taken into the contract of care, but it could be argued that the model needs redrawing to convey this.

The multidisciplinary team's role

It is important to recognise that the first person a patient usually meets in the health care setting is a nurse. For example even if the physical arrival on a hospital ward is dealt with by a housekeeper, the nurse soon becomes the chief operator in dealing with the patient: in a community home, the person with learning disability is met first by the community nurse.

Very soon in the episode of hospital care, a doctor arrives on the scene and may be followed by the physiotherapist, occupational therapist, laboratory technician, social worker etc. The normal practice is for the nurse to concentrate on the formulation of a comprehensive care plan to include aspects of physical, emotional, spiritual and social needs. Other carers in the environment also proceed to document their own perception of the needs of the patient. The documention may stay on the ward or may follow the patient out, into a department within the hospital, or into an office within the Social Services Department. This means that not only may the care plan be outside the ward and outside the hospital, but also it may be outside the premises of the Health Authority. This rather curious process unfolds with a varying degree of interaction between the professionals themselves and the patient. The result is that a number of discrete observations are made on paper, observations that may not be used or read by all in the team looking after the patient.

The concept of integrated or corporate care planning has recently been highlighted by the Audit Commission NHS (1991), which is auditing the care planning policies of all District Health Authorities in England and Wales for 1992 onwards. It will be necessary for all providers of care to demonstrate that a method of multidisciplinary care planning is implemented as part of a drive to enhance the quality of care delivered to patients. Later in the chapter the real benefits of integrated care will be addressed, but meanwhile it is necessary to illustrate how an integrated plan may be developed and what it could look like.

For purposes of clarity let us take as our example Mary Smith who has breast cancer, was admitted to a surgical ward without the benefit of prior discussion as to the nature of the surgical intervention, but has been welcomed and the necessary reassurances given by her named nurse.

Firstly, Mary Smith will be asked for her biographical details: full name and address, social and family history, etc. Ideally, such information need not be collected again during this admission by any other practitioner.

Next a series of separate assessments will be carried out by the named nurse and medical officer but, depending on what might arise from these assessments, other members may be added to the team of carers, e.g. a physiotherapist or a specialist nurse counsellor experienced in breast care. These assessments allow specific professional interests to be satisfied, but Mary Smith would be engaged as an active participant at all times. It may be possible to enlist her as a full blown member of the team encouraging her to compile her own assessment as she perceives it. A relative or advocate may in certain circumstances be nominated to act on her behalf. Each assessment might be colour coded for ease of reference. Medical assessment will include a relevant systems review and base line laboratory work. Nursing assessments will follow a different pattern but should attempt to provide a 'nursing diagnosis' rather than a formal disease-related diagnosis which is the responsibility of the medical officer.

When these assessments have been completed a multidisciplinary case conference would be held to identify and agree the problems arising. The participating professionals, in turn, will assume the lead responsibility for certain problems and discuss each one with their team colleagues so that very quickly, and without too much emphasis on the 'paper work', problems will be numbered and allocated enough space in the document for their full evaluation to be undertaken. These problems will not necessarily fall into a conventional 'nursing' pattern as some problems in Mary Smith's case will be shared. An example of a shared objective might be in the area of pre-operative counselling. The medical officer will fully engage Mary Smith in an option appraisal of appropriate treatments and then enable her, with the nurse's help, to choose the option considered to be the most appropriate. The skills of those involved in this process will be tested sorely at times as each agrees to opt in and out of the interactions as appropriate. The 'lead' person will vary from time to time and from case to case, but it is vital for the team communication to be as effective and open as possible, with the professional assuming the role of servant rather than master.

The reader may challenge the possibility of carrying out a multi-disciplinary case conference in busy acute medical and surgical wards with a very quick turnover of patients. It is probably much easier to imagine this process taking place in mental health settings, midwifery or in the community. However, the process of professionals speaking together not only depends upon their ability to gather around a bed, but also to interact through high technology which now facilitates computerised care planning and people talking together over considerable distances. In the future health care will take on the challenge which this technology brings and thus the notion of professionals getting together is made more simple. It must, however, be an axiom of care planning that technology does not rule out face-to-face interaction so necessary for personalised care, both amongst the professionals and with the patient.

All aspects of Mary Smith's care will require detailed documentation unless problems are transient and open to immediate resolution. A problem list should be drawn up to act as a 'table of contents' and 'index' combined. Once a specific problem has been resolved this is indicated on the list and new problems are added as discovered. It is important that all clinicians sign their name against the problem if it is allocated to them.

Once Mary Smith's treatment and care are under way, it is important to identify progress on a care flow sheet. All team members will use this sheet, irrespective of discipline, and will record all observations made, any additional comments and narrative, signing each one. Mary Smith may be encouraged to enter aspects of her progress as seen by herself and thus be as fully participating as her condition allows. Further sheets will be required for laboratory, X-ray and other observational records.

Finally, a discharge summary will be completed, containing brief notes of the problems encountered, information to the general practitioner and district nurse, and any recommendations for home care. The patient receives a copy of this summary and becomes the subject of a functional post-discharge audit within an agreed number of days to ensure that no aspect of care is being missed. It is probably one of the most vital aspects of Mary Smith's care that she is carefully followed up after discharge. The nature of her breast cancer, the emotional consequence of disfiguring treatment, problems relating to her sexuality and a host of other factors assume vast proportions once the patient is at home.

Currently, nurses have within this book a number of 'principles' which facilitate care planning, and care for patients with breast cancer may be found within those principles under the chapter headings of pain, dying and bereavement, expressing sexuality, learning, recreation and play, and others. Nurses could share these objectives with any relevant member of the multidisciplinary team in an effort to move towards the integration of planning and care outlined in this chapter and illustrated in *Figure 5*.

It is imperative to consider an audit process of such integrated planning in order to monitor changes in the quality outcome of episodes of care. *Figure 6* represents a diagrammatic model of how this may be carried out in connection with the 'audit square' illustrated in *Figure 1* (page 3). In the Introduction we see that the patient is not part of the planning team but is mentioned in the centre of the

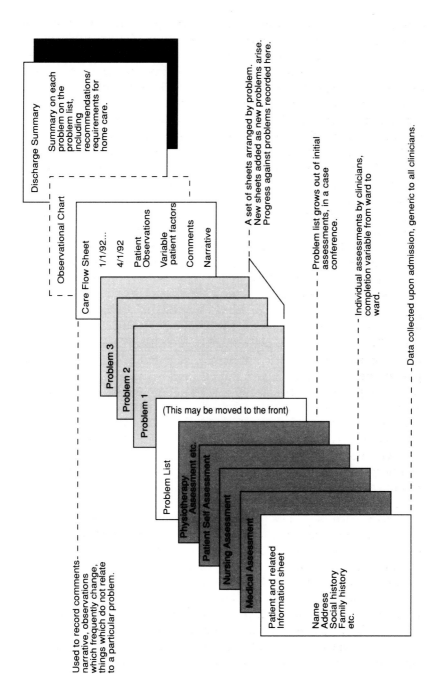

Discharge Summary

Summary on each problem on the problem list, including recommendations/ requirements for home care.

Observational Chart

Used to record comments, narrative, observations which frequently change, things which do not relate to a particular problem.

Care Flow Sheet

1/1/92...
4/1/92
Patient Observations
Variable patient factors
Comments
Narrative

Problem 3

Problem 2

Problem 1

(This may be moved to the front)

Problem List

Physiotherapy Assessment etc.

Patient Self Assessment

Nursing Assessment

Medical Assessment

Patient and related Information sheet

Name
Address
Social history
Family history
etc.

A set of sheets arranged by problem. New sheets added as new problems arise. Progress against problems recorded here.

Problem list grows out of initial assessments, in a case conference.

Individual assessments by clinicians, completion variable from ward to ward.

Data collected upon admission, generic to all clinicians.

Figure 5. Care record for single patient.

square as the subject of audit only, but not involved in that process. *Figure 6* seeks to demonstrate that the patient is fully involved in both processes of planning and audit. By such involvement of the patient the vital intelligence that she can bring to a comprehensive care plan is acknowledged, and by having fulfilled the objectives within that plan the professionals can be satisfied that they have done a good job: this is confirmed by the patient without whom neither care planning nor audit would be necessary.

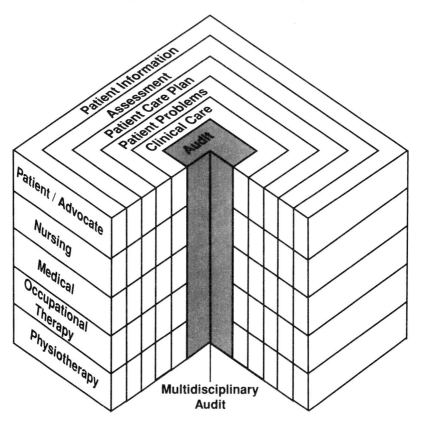

Figure 6. Audit process for integrated care planning.

Advantages of intergrated care planning

The real advantages that are likely to be gained by the patient through an integrated care planning approach are given below.

- The members of the multidisciplinary team have communicated effectively through a process of co-operative problem-solving mechanisms.

- At all stages of the patient's care, each professional involved has considered the individual contribution of others.
- Because the professionals concerned corporately 'own' the care plan, there is a creative tension within the team for each member to achieve the objectives set for the patient's benefit.
- A single record of care is more valuable in pursuit of complaint investigations in that the record does not consist of numerous isolated parts.
- Care audit can be processed more easily through group review mechanisms.
- The single record leads to a situation where the focus is on care as an integrated, shared, patient-orientated pursuit rather than on the quality of nursing care only.
- The fully participating patient/advocate feels little loss of dignity or control, is more confident and above all is in a position to maintain a sense of importance in his own affairs.

Only time will tell the story of how nurses have succeeded in influencing the direction of care. It is undeniable that nurses are in the best position of all carers to move forward in the crusade to make the patient 'king'.

References

Department of Health (1988) *New Clinical Grading Structure for Nurses Midwives and Health Visitors*, Executive Letter, p.33.

Audit Commission National Health Service (1991) *The Virtue of Patients: Making best use of ward nursing resources*, National Health Service Report No.4, London.

Index